MILE HIGH
& HEALTHY

MILE HIGH
&HEALTHY

The Frequent Traveler's Roadmap to Eating,
Energy, Exercise and a Balanced Life.

*Wishing you happy and
healthy travels!*

Jayne McAllister

JAYNE MCALLISTER, MA

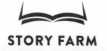

STORY FARM

Mile High and Healthy: The Frequent Traveler's Roadmap to Eating,
Energy, Exercise and a Balanced Life
© 2015 by Jayne McAllister
www.jaynemcallister.com

Published in the United States of America by Story Farm, LLC
www.story-farm.com

Library of Congress Cataloguing-in-Publication Data is available
upon request.
ISBN 978-0-9966038-2-9
Printed in Canada

Designer: Lauren Eggert
Lead editor: Scott Morris
Copy editor: Veronica Randall
Editorial assistant: Marcela Oliveira
Production management: Tina Dahl

10 9 8 7 6 5 4 3 2 1
First Edition, December 2015

For David Mulvaney, with gratitude.

TABLE OF CONTENTS

TABLE OF CONTENTS

FOREWORD

If you're one of a growing number of travelers who frequently finds yourself in an airport or airplane, on the road, rails or even in a yak cart, then *Mile High and Healthy* is a page-turning trip you need to take.

Jayne McAllister has been a self-professed "road warrior" for much of her extensive career. While reviewing this book I have grown to know her a bit better and have found her to be a person who enjoys—maybe even thrives— on the adventure of travel. I believe she has found, however, during those many years of extensive travel, that the thrill of adventure diminishes when the travel becomes a routine part of one's work.

Roald Amundsen, the esteemed Norwegian explorer and leader of the first successful expedition to the South Pole, famously crystalized this point saying: "Adventure is just bad planning." I am absolutely sure that Amundsen and all of those many participants of that arduous two-year exploration had more than their share of adventure. I am equally sure that they must have all shared the longing, the aching—at some point even the need—to just get to the South Pole as efficiently, prompt-ly (dare I write comfortably?) as humanly possible. At some point in the journey they must have just wanted to get there and get back home without adventure.

In this book, Jayne offers a unique source of information for all of those travelers who may just want to get there and get back home as efficiently as possible. This is also a treasure trove of information for those less frequent travelers, hoping for a smidgen of adventure, but wanting to minimize the joys of jet lag; traveler's diarrhea; and/or airline mismanagement during their voyage.

Jayne has worked in travel for much of her career. She has been a travel magazine publisher, logging close to two million flying miles during her work. She has been a guest speaker on Fox and ABC News as well as national radio and television talk shows as a travel wellness expert. She is the founder and man-ager of the Business Travel Wellness Conference.

I first met her as a student in my Anatomy and Physiology class at Indian River State College in Vero Beach, FL. She very quickly demonstrated a level of interest, aptitude and academ-ic authority that, quite frankly, I simply wasn't used to. Had I known that she was a Cambridge graduate with a BA and MA degree in languages, I may not have been quite as surprised at her relentless attention and studiousness but would have still been impressed.

When she asked me to review the medical and scientific accuracy of this book I was honored and genuinely interest-ed. I have always been thrilled with the planning and process of traveling. I have also traveled extensively throughout my career but more on the adventurous end of the spectrum than the "road warriors" of business world today.

I served in the United States Army for 24 years as a research physiologist and an anesthesiologist participating in travel-related research and medical treatment of our soldiers. While stationed at the U.S. Army Research Institute of Environmental Medicine in Natick, MA, we investigated factors associated with rapid deployment to extreme environmental conditions. While serving as an anesthesiologist in Afghanistan we would often have very real travel concerns related to transport of our patients.

While assuredly a bit more peripheral in the study of travel than Jayne, I have been thrilled to be associated with the writing of this very practical and useful resource, and I am confident in assuring it as a scientifically and medically reliable book.

Happy—safe and comfortable—travels.

James W. Agnew, MD, PhD

INTRODUCTION

I've been destined to travel since I was two years old and used to accompany my grandfather on work trips for British Rail. With sandwiches and a soda pop carefully packed by Grandma, I learned at an early age the cliché that it's about the journey not the destination. I would later learn that for all of the wonderful things that travel brings—experiencing other cultures, seeing new worlds and exotic people, expanding one's mind—there are some serious costs that go along with it, and some of these have nothing to do with the price of airline tickets and hotels.

Basically what I learned was this: Your mind is not the only thing that expands when you travel regularly. Let's fast-forward 20 years:

I'd graduated from Cambridge with a degree in modern languages and had spent a lot of time in France, Spain and Egypt, plus an entire year teaching English in a Sudanese government school. My sandwich and soda had been upgraded thanks to the amazing variety of food my travels afforded me. But as my horizons expanded, so did my waistline and derrière! Yes, my career grew and so did my appetite. Moving to a new country on my own, I filled the void in my personal life with food and packed on 20 pounds thanks to my nomadic existence.

Finally, I decided to go on a diet: I skipped meals, really easy to do when you're traveling. I ate cookies for breakfast, pasta for lunch, had just a glass of wine for dinner. Believe it or not, this worked, although I'd go to bed starving every night. I moved on to my "maintenance" plan of lattes and candy bars until dinner, which was often with clients (I was selling advertising for international publications). I'd order what I thought was a healthy meal and wash it down with wine and very little water.

At this point, I looked slim, but I wasn't healthy. I was in my 20s, and my idea of balancing work life and personal life was putting in 12-hour days, then meeting friends for drinks. Even at that age, such a lifestyle couldn't be sustained without consequences. I had very little energy and could barely get out of bed in the morning. Lancôme stock did great thanks to my voluminous skincare purchases, but I lost my glow anyway. My hair was dull, too. I didn't realize that my entire being had lost its sparkle. At the time, I wasn't linking my dining choices to my mental and physical states.

My wake-up call came when I was diagnosed with osteopenia. I was 39 years old, a publisher of an inflight magazine traveling through North America, Europe and the Caribbean 180 days a year. Osteopenia is the precursor to osteoporosis, the loss in bone density that leads to painful fractures and even death in elderly people. I was too young for this diagnosis.

My mother and grandmother had osteoporosis, but I'd never given it any thought. I lived in ignorant bliss under the mistaken assumption that I was "healthy." Yet here was my doctor explaining that I had the bones of someone 15 years older. If left unchecked, the dowager hump that was beginning to form would take on a whole new visual as my spine rounded over in hyper-kyphosis. Eventually, I'd be walking with a cane, terrified to sneeze in case I broke a rib. Back then Fosomax was the standard prescription, and it had vile side effects including nausea, dizziness and joint swelling.

I didn't want the illness, yet I didn't want the pharmaceutical cure, either. Surely there had to be a healthy way to overcome this. My doctor told me it would take at least two years to turn matters around on my own, at which point he would insist on the brutal medication.

As I researched the causes of bone density loss, many familiar faces showed up: alcohol, caffeine, smoking (I'd smoked in my early 20s), too much animal protein, too much dairy, and lack of weight-bearing exercise. My regimen of swimming, smoking and lattes wasn't looking too good.

I had to change. I had no choice. I sought foods that would increase my bone density and gradually changed my eating habits across the board. I cut back on alcohol. I began doing weight-bearing exercise daily no matter where I was in the world. Before long my energy increased, my eyes started to sparkle again and my skin cleared up.

Finally, I took a leap of faith and I left my corporate job to pursue my new-found passion for health and fitness. Despite living on a Caribbean island at the time, I left home, husband and cat, for a yearlong sojourn in New York City to study Pilates, integrative nutrition and transformational coaching.

The net result is that, today, my weight is stable, my sugar cravings have disappeared and I have more energy than ever. I'm able to run two businesses without undue stress. I travel frequently and when I'm not traveling, I'm planning my next trip because I miss it so much. Jet lag is nonexistent for me. I eat out all the time when I travel, and I enjoy fine wine. I sleep between eight and nine hours a night and find plenty of time for my friends, my garden and my books. I stay in shape by doing only exercise that I love.

To bring things full circle, I proved my doctor completely wrong by drastically reducing the osteopenia in my spine and eliminating it from my hip in just eight months.

It was only natural that I would want to share my hard-won knowledge of how to combine two of my greatest passions—travel and wellness. After all, I've experienced first-hand all the traps, dead ends, fads and tricks that don't work. I've spent years studying and practicing what does work, and learning how to make these techniques as convenient for the traveler as possible.

Don't worry—this doesn't mean packing kale and quinoa salad in your hand luggage or eschewing Bordeaux when you're out for dinner with clients. Being Mile High and Healthy is about having it all.

Many people assume business travelers lead a glamorous lifestyle: tooling around in first class; flying all over the world; racking up frequent flyer points; entertaining clients with fabulous dinners out; soaking up rays between meetings and, basically, barely working for a living.

Consider a more realistic scenario: You get up at 4 a.m. to make a flight that is delayed. You fly to a city for a one-day meeting because your employer is too cheap to pay for a hotel the night before. You arrive at your meeting about ready for a nap yet anxious to make a good impression, so you're fired up on caffeine and cookies. You skipped lunch because there was no meal service on the plane, and you had to sprint through the airport at record speeds to make it to your meeting on time.

With the meeting concluded, you check into your hotel 30 minutes before your business dinner. You barely have time to clean up, never mind rest or exercise. Half a bottle of claret and too much rich, expense-account food later, you crawl into bed. Sleep eludes you thanks to indigestion, the noise of the ice machine, and the snoring of the guest in the next room.

And you realize you forgot to call home...

On top of this, there is the toll of being away from home and missing important family events. This is far from the picture of health.

Mile High and Healthy is about having the energy to get through just such a day without crashing and burning. It allows you to make the best dining choices available to you wherever you are. You will learn how to get eight hours of uninterrupted sleep and how to stick to a consistent exercise program wherever you are on the planet. All of which will be vital when it comes to keeping relationships with loved ones on an even keel even if you're not there for the biggest successes and emergencies. It's about having the wherewithal to juggle eight balls at once but to have fun while you're doing so.

Each chapter of this book addresses a particular challenge faced by road warriors the world over. You can dip into selected sections if you need specific information. That said, most frequent travelers are A types, so enjoy the full gamut as you go from cover to cover. *Mile High and Healthy* will show you how to:

★ Eat the right foods on the run.

★ Exercise consistently, even in a plane, train, automobile or your typical shoebox of a Parisian hotel room.

★ Defy circumstances and enjoy sufficient sleep.

★ Find time for relaxation that doesn't include surfing the web.

★ Choose how to handle stress.

★ Wave goodbye to jet lag.

★ Stay lovingly connected with family and friends.

★ Maintain a strong immune system.

Sound like a tall order? Follow the steps in this book and you'll find yourself on the road to optimum health and to having it all.

// DOES THIS SOUND LIKE YOU? //

★You have a hard time losing or maintaining weight on the road because you're eating out so often and/or entertaining clients frequently.

★When your weight goes up, you spend all your time trying to compensate for it when you get home.

★Every day you try to include exercise in your schedule but it gets crowded out because you have an early start, you're in meetings or on a plane.

★It takes all you have to muster enough energy to get through your day.

★Jet lag wipes you out for days, and you can never get on the right time schedule.

★You feel like the Michelin Man—your belly has puffed up and your feet are swollen—after every trip, you have more gas than the Goodyear Blimp.

★You spend your spare time working.

★You spend more time with your phone than your family.

★The concept of self-care is completely alien to you, as is the subtle art of being able to say "no."

CHAPTER 1

HEALTHY EATING
ON THE ROAD

//PREPARE TO TAKEOFF//

"Excess weight. Spiking blood sugar. Fatigue due to airport junk food. This chapter provides the tools to help you lose the things that are keeping you down."

The frequent traveler is a survivor, a model of efficiency and a master of adaptation. You can spot one in an airport instantly. They are usually more formally dressed than other travelers. They appear confident—they know where they are, where they're going and how to get there as gracefully and efficiently as possible. Next to these road warriors, almost everybody else appears to be an amateur.

But beneath the professional façade, a dark secret lurks. I know that secret. I'm in the business of helping hard-working, globetrotting, high-achievers, and they come to me, sometimes bordering on desperation, with a secret. The secret is they feel the opposite of how they appear. They *are* the opposite of how they appear.

If you are one of them, I know why you're reading this: You're exhausted, sapped, brittle, nursing digestive discomfort and back pain, fighting weight gain, heaping long-term damage on your body and soul due to your brutal schedule. You feel powerless against the many bad habits bred by travel.

Mile High and Healthy has the answers you need, from diet to exercise to contending with that chronically aching back. But let's start with the questions I'm usually asked first:

How the heck do I eat healthily on the road? What am I supposed to do when there seem to be no healthy options and I'm stuck at an airport?

How can I eat healthily when it's all Continental breakfasts at hotels and fast food on the run?

And those enormous meals with clients at expensive restaurants where the wine flows like tap water and the usual menu amounts to a tempting list of buttered starches and fatty meats—how can I stay fit and increase my energy eating under those circumstances?

The answers to these questions ultimately involve all the other chapters as well as this one, as *Mile High and Healthy* embraces a holistic approach. Still, food is the best place to start the discussion. Food is visceral. It is delicious. We can't actually live without it. And it is a time-honored comfort. In fact, food sometimes seems like the only consolation when you're hitting three cities and six meetings in two days. Hello, gourmet cheeseburger!

Just hold on a minute. Back away from the friendly, airport gastro-pub with craft beers and half-pound Angus burgers with exotic aiolis and hand-cut French fries. Read on. I'm going to dive in with some specific strategies for dealing with the difficulty of maintaining a healthy diet on the road, and then later in the chapter I'll lay out some general nutrition principles applicable in any time zone, in any airport, any time of the day or night.

Healthy eating can be an elusive specter for the frequent traveler: You grab the first thing you see as you dash through an airport, deal with a badly planned schedule that gives you no time to eat or discover there's no meal service onboard, attend a business breakfast and lunch that serves donuts and pizza respectively and, finally, end your day with a heavy and very late dinner.

"...FOOD SOMETIMES SEEMS LIKE THE ONLY CONSOLATION WHEN YOU'RE HITTING THREE CITIES AND SIX MEETINGS IN TWO DAYS. HELLO, GOURMET CHEESEBURGER! JUST HOLD ON A MINUTE. BACK AWAY FROM THE FRIENDLY, AIRPORT GASTRO-PUB WITH CRAFT BEERS AND HALF-POUND ANGUS BURGERS WITH EXOTIC AIOLIS. READ ON. I'M GOING TO DIVE IN WITH SOME SPECIFIC STRATEGIES FOR DEALING WITH THE DIFFICULTY OF MAINTAINING A HEALTHY DIET ON THE ROAD..."

In this scenario, there's no planning ahead and shopping accordingly. But you can make healthy choices based on what's available to you at that moment, whether you're in a hotel, airport or a catered business meeting.

In 2012, global travel company Carlson Wagonlit conducted a study of Stress Triggers for Business Travelers. The three highest ranking stressors—out of 100—were lost or delayed baggage (79/100), poor Internet connection at destination (77/100) and flying economy on medium or long-haul flights (73/100), with delays a close fourth (72/100).

"HAVING A PLAN MEANS WHEN YOU'RE FACED WITH A LACK OF CHOICES, YOU CAN DIG INTO YOUR BAG OF MILE HIGH AND HEALTHY TRICKS AND MAKE A CONFIDENT CHOICE AROUND YOUR EATING WITHOUT IT EATING AWAY AT YOU."

The same study reported that not being able to eat healthily scored 62 out of 100, higher than traveling on weekends, flying indirect versus direct and jet lag. What these factors have in common is a lack of control. In other words, frequent travelers are most fazed when they do not have control of their environment, including lack of healthy dining options.

But there's hope—frequent travelers are really good at planning, and usually have a plan B because plan A has a habit of going awry at a moment's notice. Having a plan means when you're faced with a lack of choices, you can dig into your bag of *Mile High and Healthy* tricks and make a confident choice around your eating without it eating away at you.

// PUTTING IT INTO PRACTICE
A DAY IN THE LIFE OF A TRAVELER //

Knowledge is one thing, putting it into practice is another. Here are some situations that frequent travelers face every day followed by the *Mile High and Healthy* way of handling them.

AT THE AIRPORT

First of all, you may have noticed things are getting better in terms of airport food options. There's been a revolution over the last few years as restaurants associated with celebrity chefs keep popping up worldwide: Gordon Ramsay's Plane Food at Heathrow Terminal 5; Todd English's Bonfire at Boston's Logan International and JFK; Tyler Florence's Rotisserie at San Francisco; and Charles Gaig's Michelin-starred Porta Gaig at Barcelona's El Prat.

These aren't necessarily healthy eating establishments per se, but if the quality of ingredients is elevated (less processed and fresher), that's a huge step forward. Take Vino Volo, for example—yes, it's a wine bar located in over 20 airports in the US and Canada (in multiple terminals in some instances), but where there's an effort to pour decent wine, food offerings tend to be more thoughtful. Vino Volo's menu contains several healthy options, and half portions of many dishes are available.

Food trucks offer an interesting dining option. Usually located in cell phone lots, you'll find food trucks at Austin, Tampa, Cincinnati, Tucson, and San Francisco airports. Cuisines are varied, but most deliver locally sourced fresh food, plus you know there's a fast turnover on ingredients. But keep away from hot dog and bakery-themed trucks.

Each November, the Physicians' Committee for Responsible Medicine releases its Airport Food Review. This handy round-up ranks the 30 busiest US airports according to their restaurants with the healthiest menu options, based on entrees featuring vegetables, fruits, whole grains and legumes.

The 2014 Review reported, "Seventy-five percent of restaurants at 23 of the top 30 busiest US airports offer at least one healthful, plant-based entrée." Of course, you're going to have to hope that if there is only one single solitary healthy dish, it's available in your terminal.

On the other hand, you might be lucky enough to be flying out of San Francisco International where Tastes On The Fly brought the local dining scene to the airport, including the award-winning Napa Farms Market and, more recently, opened the Berkshire Farms Market at Boston's Logan International.

Today's traveler has multiple resources at their fingertips. You can check out in advance what is available in your terminal and pull up menus online. For example, the sandwich chain Au Bon Pain posts menus for each of their airport locations on their website. You can learn such useful information as the roast beef herbed cheese sandwich has 150 fewer calories than the chicken avocado, and they have a veggie and hummus wrap that packs a whopping 15 grams of fiber. Taking a few minutes to research what's available in your location and order a meal in advance keeps you in control of both your time and your waistline.

If you have the budgetary option to skip the food court and head for a "real" restaurant, please do. By real restaurant, I mean an establishment that cooks food to order compared with fast-food joints that precook and preassemble their offerings. This makes it infinitely easier for you to order with healthy modifications, such as hold the mayo, skip the cheese or broiled rather than fried.

The onus is on you to do the homework, but you should only need to do it once for each destination. You'll get to the point where you can look forward to dining at Reagan National Airport's Legal Seafoods and enjoying the Swordfish Kabob with Quinoa.

"REDUCING FOOD TO A NUMBER IS AN UNHEALTHY OBSESSION. AS LONG AS YOU EAT A VARIETY OF UNPRO-CESSED FOODS, YOU'LL ACHIEVE THE RIGHT BALANCE OF NUTRIENTS."

8 TIPS
FOR EATING HEALTHILY AT AN AIRPORT FOOD COURT

Sometimes airport food courts might be the only option that your budget and schedule allow. Nowadays they range from the sublime to the ridiculous, from cinnamon rolls to Tortas Frontera at Chicago O'Hare. Renowned local chef Rick Bayless offers freshly made guacamole, homemade chips and salsa plus a bunch of different tortas. Bayless even lists the local farms from which the meat is purveyed.

But that's the food court exception. Then there's the real world for the rest of us. We're in the terminal that's offering pseudo-Chinese and hotdogs. What to do?

1 // If you're stuck for healthy choices, aim for simple. My favorite trio of soup, salad and sandwich can be tracked down pretty much anywhere. Of course there are caveats, like no cheese and beer soup, Caesar salads or cheesy meatball subs.

2 // Your salad should have an oil-based dressing and no croutons. Choose as many vegetables as possible, especially greens. Romaine tops iceberg nutritionally. Look for spinach and kale, too.

3 // Your sandwich should be on whole grain bread. Tuna and chicken salad in mayonnaise are out. Slices of lean meat are in. Less is more—no need to have meat and cheese, you only need one of the two for fat and protein. Always sneak in at least one veggie serving to your sandwich, even if it's lettuce or a slice of tomato. Choose mustard over mayonnaise.

4 // Soups are an excellent option as long as they're not full of milk and cream. Choose soups with vegetables and beans or lentils for fiber and energy. Whatever you order will probably have a lot of salt in it, so drink lots of water to flush it out before you fly.

5 // For Asian food court offerings, look for a vegetable dish, rice noodles, fish or a simple combo like chicken and broccoli. Ask that your dish be made to order without salt or MSG. Request less soy and oil. Always ask for brown rice, although it might not be available. If you can't avoid starch-laden white rice, order a protein with your veggies, that way your blood sugar won't spike as much. Miso soup and noodles in broth are good choices, but skip teriyaki because it's both very salty and sugary.

6 // Sushi bars can be good options. Even if only white rice is available, the protein and seaweed will offset the effects of the starch. Be warned: It's easy to get carried away calorie-wise with sushi. Each piece is between 50 and 60 calories. Sushi rolls are around 300 calories, assuming there are no batter-fried ingredients, like tempura.

7 // Smoothie bars are popping up in airports now. Tread cautiously: Many chain smoothie bars use packaged (meaning processed) juices with lots of hidden sugars. Take the time to read the ingredients even if you have to get to the airport five minutes sooner!

8 // Most airports have a Mexican eatery that have great options if you skip the cheese. Black beans, rice (preferably brown), guacamole, fresh salsa and a corn tortilla provide protein, carbohydrates and healthy fats.

INFLIGHT DINING

Inflight dining can be very grim. According to Nikos Loukas, CEO of inflightfeed.com and a consultant to the airline catering industry, most economy class airline meals are made anywhere from three to 18 months in advance. Yes, I'll repeat: most economy class airline meals are made anywhere from three to 18 months in advance.

If you want fresher food and you're stuck in steerage, order a special meal. I particularly recommend ordering vegan, even if you're an omnivore, because you'll have a meal that is higher in fiber, vegetable content, and lower in saturated fat, all of which help prevent inflight bloating.

According to Loukas, special meals are made closer to flying time, quite often the same day, just like business and first class meals. Special meal options vary according to the airline, but to give you an idea, British Airways offers Lacto Ovo Vegetarian, Vegan, Asian Vegetarian, Hindu, Muslim, Kosher, Diabetic, Gluten Intolerant, Low Calorie, Low Fat, Low Salt and Low Lactose.

At the other end of the spectrum is Korean Air, which has its own organic farms, raising cattle and poultry as well as vegetables, including hydroponic tomatoes and peppers. However, you only get the grass-fed beef in premium classes. (Check out http://www.cntraveler.com/galleries/2013-06-11/photos-korean-air-farm for more information about the farm).

One option for economy class is to preorder for upgraded meals if the airline offers this service. Air France has a fantastic à la carte service in economy and premium economy classes, offering fresh, seasonal items. Menus range from €12 to €28 euros. (Prices were accurate when this book went to press, but are subject to change.)

Singapore Airlines, whose meal service is renowned, lets

premium economy and above classes preselect their meals through its Book the Cook Advance Meal Selection Service. There is no charge for Book the Cook, and there is a wide variety of dishes to choose from (over 60 out of Singapore), so taking advantage of this service will ensure the healthiest options available to you. On flights to London, lighter selections include Oriental Marinated Fish with Fried Rice, Vegetarian Stew with Couscous and Thai Green Chicken Curry. To Paris, pick from Roasted Cod with Wild Rice, Masala Shrimp and Basil Chicken and Thai Rice (there is also fattening French fare but I'll ignore that).

As far as purchasing food onboard, you might be able to find something fresh and healthy amid the aging, processed options. For example, Delta Airlines has partnered with Luvo Inc., the Washington state-based company that delivers prepared foods with antibiotic-free meat and poultry and nonGMO ingredients whenever possible. Fresh snacks, salads and wraps (under 500 calories) are available on select flights.

Air Canada Café offers several items for purchase, including a fresh spinach salad, sushi bento box, hummus and pretzels, and celery and carrots with ranch dip. Flight length and destination determine menu offerings.

> "INFLIGHT DINING CAN BE VERY GRIM. ACCORDING TO NIKOS LOUKAS, CEO OF INFLIGHTFEED.COM AND A CONSULTANT TO THE AIRLINE CATERING INDUSTRY, MOST ECONOMY CLASS AIRLINE MEALS ARE MADE ANYWHERE FROM THREE TO 18 MONTHS IN ADVANCE."

Clearly all airline food is not created equal, so your best bet is to check the airline's website for special meal options and preordering services.

Consider taking your own food from home onboard, or pick up something easily transportable before you board. Having healthy food with you at all times eradicates excuses and keeps you in charge of your dining choices. Rule

Number One, be fair to the passengers around you and do not take stinky food onboard. That means no burgers, fries, tuna salad or sandwiches, or bean burritos.

If you're worried about not having enough time to select and collect your meal while dashing through the terminal, enter the AirGrub app that allows you to book food for preflight pick-up. Simply search by airport or flight information, order your meal based on the options available in your terminal, and once there, skip the line and pick up your meal. If your flight plans go awry, AirGrub customer service will cancel your order and refund your purchase.

AirGrub launched in 2015 at San Francisco Airport and will be rolled out at other major US airports soon.

AT A RESTAURANT

Okay, so you're eating out between two and three times a day. That's up to 15 opportunities in a working week to eat larger portions and to ingest more salt, sugar and saturated fat than you likely would at home.

You may also experience a strange phenomenon that I call Menu Zoning. This is when you open the menu and instantly forget good intentions. You come to the restaurant ready to have your salad plus grilled fish and veggies, then you open the menu and all bets are off. Your eyes glaze over, and all you can see are the fried calamari and fettucine Alfredo jumping out at you. Before you know it, you've wolfed said squid and pasta, as well as two thirds of the bread basket (buttered, of course!) and a tiramisu. You order things you wouldn't dream of touching at home, and you order lots of them.

THE BEST WAYS TO AVOID MENU ZONING ARE:

★ **Use process of elimination.** Once you have an open menu in front of you, start by mentally eliminating all unsuitable items. That means anything with the words "cream," "fried," "cheese" or all three.

★ **Start your meal with soup** (noncreamy). You'll consume 20 percent fewer calories and will feel full enough not to overeat for the rest of the meal.

★ **Check out the menu online beforehand.** Don't be too swayed by the specials unless they are healthy choices.

Another rule of thumb is to be prepared to be a PITA, or pain-in-the-ass. You might feel uncomfortable being "that person" when ordering out, but you can do it with grace and discretion. If you have genuine dietary issues, such as being gluten or lactose intolerant, it's fair to call the restaurant in advance (if you have that opportunity) and ask if they will make substitutions. Nowadays restaurants are more used than ever to accommodating patrons with special diets.

The key is to be prepared to ask for what you want. For example, can the meat or fish be grilled rather than fried? Can an extra vegetable be substituted for the starch? How many vegetables can they rustle up for you? Can the fish or steak be served over asparagus instead of pasta?

Some establishments won't make any substitutions. In that case, hopefully they're thoughtful enough to provide healthy options, such as lean proteins and steamed vegetables, with any rich, heavy sauces served on the side.

Basically, a healthy diet starts with eating more vegetables, fewer processed foods and fewer animal proteins. Your number-one goal when eating in a restaurant is to add as many vegetables to your meal as possible to balance out the less healthy items.

TIPS FOR FIGHTING FAT WITH VEGGIES

1 // Crowd out the bad guys by adding in vegetables. Crowding out doesn't mean eliminating everything else on your plate. By eating more vegetables, you'll simply consume less animal protein and more fiber.

2 // Have a salad before each meal to curb your appetite and ensure that you consume a slew of micronutrients, whether you care about that or not. Dress your salad to ensure absorption of the micronutrients in the vegetables via the fat.

3 // The salad dressing should consist of olive oil and freshly squeezed lemon juice or vinegar. Creamy dressings are a no-no. Olive oil contains "good" oils, including essential and monounsaturated, which are heart-healthy. When dressing your own salad, stick to about a tablespoonful. If you can get your salad predressed, please do, as it's more likely to have the right amount on it.

4 // Substitute extra vegetables for starchy potatoes and white rice.

5 // Create your own entrée with side dishes, choosing lots of veggies to fill your plate and your stomach.

As for protein choices, keep your order as simple as possible to limit opportunities for hidden calories and fatty ingredients to lurk. Simple cuts of meat or fish with raw or steamed veggies are the best way to go.

Beware of the myth of choosing chicken over beef to cut down on saturated fat. Dr. Neal Barnard of the Physicians' Committee for Responsible Medicine reminds us that the leanest cut of beef is 28 percent fat while the leanest part of chicken is 24 percent fat.

Pick good starches, such as brown rice, quinoa and barley, just limit your portion to half a cup and mix with veggies for a high-fiber, low-calorie serving. Politely decline the bread.

Beware huge pasta servings. When were you ever served the recommended two ounces dry weight? Let's face it, you'd probably have a fit if such a paltry amount were served to you in a restaurant. That's how accustomed we are to overeating.

A pound of pasta is cheap so throwing half a pound or more onto a plate is a great way for a restaurant to look generous and still make a decent profit margin, to which they are entitled.

The best sauces are the simplest, such as marinara or primavera. Having protein with the pasta will help temper sugar surges caused by the refined carbohydrates. Seafood either sautéed or in a red sauce is an excellent choice. Avoid creamy and heavy meat sauces.

Portion control generally can be an issue for frequent flyers because who knows when you're going to eat again? Add to that the stress of travel, which creates strong urges to find comfort in food. I can pretty much guarantee that you will not starve if you eat only half of your meal and give it time to digest. By eating lightly and digesting properly, you will feel better, sleep better, have less inflight bloating and suffer fewer effects of jetlag when you are crossing time zones.

The increase in restaurant portion sizes is a problem facing anyone who dines out frequently, not just travelers. In 2002, Marion Nestle and Lisa Young of New York University pub-

> "PORTION CONTROL CAN BE AN ISSUE FOR FREQUENT FLYERS BECAUSE YOU MIGHT THINK YOU NEED TO EAT EVERYTHING IN FRONT OF YOU IF YOU DON'T KNOW WHEN YOU'RE GOING TO EAT AGAIN. ADD TO THAT THE FACT THAT THE STRESS OF TRAVEL CREATES STRONG URGES TO FIND COMPENSATION IN THE COMFORT OF FOOD."

lished their important findings about portion sizes in *The American Journal of Public Health*. They reported that portion sizes "have been rising since the 1970's, rose sharply in the 1980s, and have continued in parallel with increasing body weights."

A 2003 study from the University of Pennsylvania compared portion sizes at similar establishments in France and the US, concluding that the average meal in France is 25 percent smaller than in America. That may go a long way to demystifying the French Paradox of rich foods and svelte bodies.

The study's author, Paul Rozin, explains: "Many studies have shown that, if food is moderately palatable, people tend to consume what is put in front of them and generally consume more when offered more food. Much discussion of the 'obesity epidemic' in the US has focused on personal willpower, but our study shows that the environment also plays an important role, and that people may be satisfied even if served less than they would normally eat."

Years later, little has changed. In fact, "generous" portions are not limited to entrees, but apply equally to appetizers and desserts. Consider ordering two appetizers instead of an appetizer and an entrée to keep calories down and avoid wasting leftovers, which you can't really take from a business meal anyway.

It might be time to add a little spice to your life. My absolute favorite trick is to order dishes with bold flavors—think strong spices and hot curries. Research shows that diners are more easily sated, and thus consume less, when eating flavorful rather than bland foods. Spicy cuisine awakens the taste buds and

> "IT MIGHT BE TIME TO ADD A LITTLE SPICE TO YOUR LIFE. MY ABSOLUTE FAVORITE TRICK IS TO ORDER DISHES WITH BOLD FLAVORS—THINK STRONG SPICES AND HOT CURRIES. RESEARCH SHOWS THAT DINERS ARE MORE EASILY SATED, AND THUS CONSUME LESS, WHEN EATING FLAVORFUL RATHER THAN BLAND FOODS."

//EGG-SACTLY RIGHT!//

Eggs deserve a special mention as the comeback kids of healthy eating. Long maligned for their fat and cholesterol content, studies have reported that eggs are in fact a pretty good source of nutrients, including antioxidants and vitamins A, D and E, which are "fat soluble" vitamins and are better digested with the fat in the yolk.

This means the good stuff is in the yolks! So after years of people eating tasteless egg whites in the name of good health, we now know that it's much better to eat the whole egg rather than just the albumen (the white), which is pure protein. Eggs start to lose their nutrients if they are overcooked and the yolk oxidizes, depleting antioxidant properties by about 50 percent. So, hard-boiled, fried and scrambled eggs are best avoided, and definitely forget microwaving, which reduces nutrients even more.

Many hotels offer a vat of overcooked scrambled eggs as part of a free breakfast. This gives you a difficult choice because the other available items are likely to be sugary. If you have an omelet, make sure that it contains plenty of veggies, and give it a dash of hot sauce to counter the effects of the oxidization. If you can, order your eggs soft-boiled, soft-poached or sunny-side up to keep the yolks runny. Raw eggs are the absolute best as long as they are pastured, but you'll rarely find raw offered unless you're having steak tartare, in which case please probe the server as to the eggs' quality.

In terms of quality, free-range or "pastured" eggs (eggs from hens that are free-range or pastured) are the most nutritious; they have less cholesterol, less saturated fat and more vitamin A, E, omega-3 fatty acid and beta-carotene. Better quality restaurants are serving organic and even pastured eggs, but conventional eggs are still found more widely. These are still nutritious but more likely to contain bacteria, such as salmonella, from the way they are handled.

the other senses, so you are more aware of how much you are eating and when you are full. Switching hot sauce for ketchup is a good idea because hot sauces are usually lower in calories, plus hot peppers have many health benefits.

Eat fat, fiber and protein at every meal. Combining the right foods at each meal makes for a satisfied body and mind, with fewer cravings and less overeating.

"THE TRUTH IS, JUST A LITTLE TASTE MAY BE ENOUGH TO SATE YOU. I SUGGEST HAVING THREE BITES OF DESSERT AND SAVORING EVERY MORSEL. ENJOY YOUR TREAT, THEN BE DONE AND MOVE ON WITHOUT REMORSE."

Dessert really doesn't have much place in a healthy eating program. But life is short, and there will be times you'll want to indulge. Depending on the restaurant you could find yourself faced with a mountain of chocolate mousse that would feed an army. The truth is, just a little taste is probably enough to sate you. I suggest having three bites and savoring every morsel. Enjoy your treat, then be done and move on without remorse.

BUSINESS MEALS (THE RESTAURANT TIPS APPLY HERE TOO) AND ENTERTAINING

Many of my clients work in a sales or business development capacity, which means entertaining their customers. Fostering social relationships in a convivial atmosphere is crucial to closing many deals—and usually means several courses of heavy food. It also means the ensuing digestive issues, weight gain and lack of sleep.

8 TIPS
FOR BEING THE BOSS AT BUSINESS MEALS

1 // Pick the restaurant, if possible, so you can choose somewhere with healthy options.

2 // Feeling shy about having a healthier plate than everyone else at the table? No one should be prying into your eating habits at a business meal and if they do, you might even win a convert.

3 // Beware the dining partner who is looking for an excuse to rack up their expense account (or yours) and is bent on overordering, especially expensive wine. You do not have to join them.

4 // To avoid overeating, keep your preprandial liquor intake light so you don't overindulge at dinner. Alcohol is a huge appetite stimulant.

5 // Have sparkling water with lemon to keep your water intake up.

6 // Wine goes best with food, so wait until the meal has been served before you have a glass. Make sure to consume a glass of water (or two) for each glass of wine. Savoring your beverage should mean fewer empty calories. That way, you can perhaps enjoy a better quality drink in moderation. Remember Goethe's famous words, "Life is too short to drink cheap wine."

7 // Avoid drinks with high-calorie soda mixers and opt for spirits mixed with zero-calorie soda water instead.

8 // It's easy to be distracted in a social setting and forget how much you're eating when you are engrossed in conversation. The flip side is that you might eat less if you're enjoying the conversation. So just be aware.

AT A HOTEL

Two main tips here. One is to always request a mini-fridge in your room so you can keep breakfast and snack items on hand. If you can't get a fridge, an ice bucket full of ice will keep yogurt, fruit and dips like hummus or guacamole fresh overnight.

If you're in a full service hotel that has an elaborate breakfast buffet with "everything" on it, from tropical fruits to an egg station to every bread and pastry imaginable, practice restraint. You'll find healthy options (a made-to-order veggie-filled omelet is a decent choice), but you may be sorely tempted to over eat. Don't.

At some point you may have to address the issue of your employer's travel policy. Will your company put you up at a hotel whose rooms have kitchenettes so you can prepare your own meals? Can you book, (or ask whoever books your trips to book), a property that is located close to a Whole Foods or similar store? Will they find you a hotel that has a travel wellness service in place? That way you won't have to search for better workout facilities and healthier dining options.

ROOM SERVICE

According to a 2014 report by MarketWatch, more and more hotels are removing room service from their roster of services. In the event that you do have the option to dine in your room, the same rules apply as for restaurant dining, with a couple of factors to consider.

First, remember that not all food travels well. Keep your order simple, as you don't know how long your meal will be sitting before it gets to you. (That's why eggs are usually a bad idea.)

Be specific when you order and make sure tempting extras aren't brought to your room. For example, inquire if rolls or breadsticks come with the meal, and if so, request that they be omitted.

IN A MEETING

Another complaint I hear from clients is the lack of healthy fare usually offered at business meetings. Trapping people in a room for hours without natural light and nothing but doughy, dairy-laden or sugary carbs to nosh on is not a recipe for productivity, and yet donuts and pizza are often the alimentation of choice at these events.

In this day and age of widespread food intolerances and special diets, one would expect to be asked about dietary issues and preferences in advance. If that's the case, don't hesitate to pipe up.

If you can eat before you go, then all the better, but that may not be practical. Take healthy snacks with you so that you can supplement or replace whatever is on offer.

If your company is hosting the meeting, don't be afraid to speak with whoever is ordering the food. I guarantee that you won't be the only one looking for healthier options.

COFFEE SHOP

A visit to the coffee shop will yield a sugar fest of baked goods and milky drinks that will have your energy levels on a

"ANOTHER COMPLAINT I HEAR FROM CLIENTS IS THE LACK OF HEALTHY FOOD THAT IS USUALLY OFFERED AT MEETINGS. STICKING PEOPLE IN A ROOM FOR HOURS WITHOUT NATURAL LIGHT AND WITH SUGARY CARBS TO NOSH ON IS NOT A RECIPE FOR PRODUCTIVITY, BUT DONUTS AND PIZZA ARE OFTEN THE ALIMENTATION OF CHOICE AT THESE EVENTS."

day-long roller coaster.

Your best bets are herbal teas, oatmeal and fruit. Beware premade packaged sandwiches. I asked at my local chain coffee shop how often they make theirs and learned that from bread board to display case is about three days. Anything edible that hangs around that long will lose its nutrients. That in turn means empty calories that will have you running on empty, too.

BEST SNACKS

Always, always have food on hand. Here are my absolute favorite travel snacks:

> "SAVORY GRANOLA IS VERY ADDICTIVE IF YOU CAN FIND IT, OTHERWISE THERE'S A VERY EASY RECIPE ON MY WEBSITE, HTTP://WWW.JAYNEM-CALLISTER.COM/SAVORY-GRANOLA."

★ Seaweed snacks weigh nothing, so I keep a packet in my handbag. Seaweed is a super food and good quality protein, making it excellent for leveling blood sugar. A whole packet is only 60 calories. Just be sure to check your teeth afterwards for green bits.

★ Sachets of nut butters to spread on brown rice cakes or apples. Go beyond peanut and try walnut, almond and cashew butters.

★ Fresh fruit has fiber and water, which will help you avoid inflight dehydration.

★ Nuts, particularly almonds or pistachios. I carry a bag with me at all times in case disaster (i.e. hunger) strikes. Around 21 almonds equals an ounce, and that should more than suffice for a snack.

★ Hummus is an excellent blend of protein, fat and fiber. It's found in many airport stores. You can also bring hummus from home. Be aware that technically it counts as a liquid and should be stored in a container smaller than 3.4 ounces in order to go through airport security.

★ Sachets of miso soup to which you add hot water.

★ A whole-wheat pita pocket stuffed with dressed greens is an easy way to transport salad.

★ Whole-grain salad made from brown rice or quinoa is robust and filling. Just make sure there's no raw onion or garlic in it if it's going to travel, because they become more pungent with time, and there's a risk of botulism from the garlic.

★ Savory granola is very addictive if you can find it, otherwise there's a very easy recipe on my website, http://www.jaynem-callister.com/savory-granola.

★ Organic sweet potato chips. These are so much better than the processed snacks you may (or may not) get on board. I'm partial to Late July's products. www.latejuly.com.

★ Raw veggies. Looking for crunch? Get adventurous. Carrots and celery are yummy, but find your inner radical and bring slices of fennel, jicama and radish with you. Even better with the hummus!

★ Chips and salsa—of course! Salsa is made from fresh, raw vegetables. Pair with gluten-free chips such as Late July (mentioned above) or lentil chips (www.mediterraneansnackfoods.com).

★ Beef jerky is very portable and handy for meat lovers.

Now that you know some practical strategies, let's take a look at some general principles of nutrition. For all of the information out there, it can be really confusing. Trends change faster than Kim Kardashian's wardrobe.

THE SKINNY: WHAT IS HEALTHY FOOD?

Healthy food is made with ingredients that are as close to their original state as possible. This means that they are rarely found in packages, and they have nothing added to them. "The healthiest food in the supermarket is the quietest food. It has no health claims," said Michael Pollan, author of *Food Rules: An Eater's Manual*, during the Food Revolution Summit, April 2015.

Eating healthily means consuming a balance and variety of macronutrients (protein, fat and carbohydrate) and micronutrients (vitamins and minerals). Unless you're on a special diet recommended by your doctor, there is no need to count carbs, calories or fat grams. Reducing food to a number is an unhealthy obsession. As long as you eat a variety of unprocessed foods, you'll achieve the right balance of nutrients.

Let's start with macronutrients. Protein became the darling of popular nutritional lore when animal protein diets leapt into the limelight with the Atkins, and more recently, Paleo diets. Americans tend to eat a lot of protein anyway, usually as meat protein. In fact, we eat between 132 and 276 pounds of meat per person per year. By and large, Americans are not educated to think in terms of plant protein yet, even though 90 percent of the world's population derives its protein from plants. Vegetable protein has the added benefit of dietary fiber, which is often lacking when the main emphasis of a meal is meat. How many restaurants serve sensibly sized meat portions and two or three vegetables (as opposed to one veg and a starch)? You're much more likely to find a huge steak, fries and onion rings.

Even the American Dietetic Association has decided that you can derive sufficient protein from plant sources. So consider experimenting with plant proteins of which good sources are beans, lentils, tofu, leafy green vegetables and whole grains.

Excessive protein consumption does have negative side effects, including osteoporosis, kidney disease and possibly some cancers. Some of these effects can be countered by the antioxidants and phytochemicals found in plant foods.

Am I telling you to go vegan? No. I'm suggesting a varied diet that includes plant proteins. As you introduce more vegetable proteins, you will benefit from the increased fiber and the immune system-boosting nutrients in the plants. As a traveler, this will lead to less likelihood of getting sick on the road, easier recovery from jet lag and better sleep.

The next macronutrient, fat, was demonized in the 1980s. As we were told to adopt low-fat diets, food manufacturers jumped at the opportunity to replace relatively expensive fat with low-cost sugar during processing. Ironically, although Americans were "dieting" by avoiding fat, they were in fact eating 300 calories more per day and getting fatter. Vestiges of the low-fat mentality remain today even as the beneficial aspects of good fat have been discovered. Now we know that certain types of fat are good for the heart and brain, but the variety of fats can be confusing and opinions in the nutrition community vary. In a nutshell, omega-3 and omega-9 fatty acids, monounsaturated fatty acids and polyunsaturated fatty acids are good

> "TODAY'S TRAVELER HAS MULTIPLE RESOURCES AT THEIR FINGER-TIPS. YOU CAN CHECK OUT IN ADVANCE WHAT IS AVAILABLE IN YOUR TERMINAL AND PULL UP MENUS ONLINE. FOR EXAMPLE, THE SANDWICH CHAIN AU BON PAIN POSTS MENUS FOR EACH OF THEIR AIRPORT LOCATIONS ON THEIR WEBSITE."

for you. Saturated fat and omega-6 are okay in small amounts. Trans fats are definitely out.

How does that translate into identifiable comestibles? Get good fats from the original sources as much as possible with small amounts from the bottle. The original sources are nuts, olives, avocadoes, oily fish, free-range poultry and eggs, and grass-fed meat. The bottle would be olive oil, flax seed oil and nut oils, with limited amounts of coconut oil and butter—never margarine. This will be an issue with restaurant dining because you won't know what quality of oil they're using. You might have to grill (pardon the pun) your server for more information.

> "SUGAR IS THE ROOT OF ALL EVIL BECAUSE IT IS HIGHLY ACIDIC AND VERY ADDICTIVE, WITH PROFOUND EFFECTS ON ENERGY AND MOOD. EXCESS SUGAR IS STORED IN THE BODY AS FAT. NEXT TIME YOU REACH FOR A LOW FAT COOKIE, TAKE HEED THAT THE FAT DOESN'T MAKE YOU FAT, THE SUGAR DOES."

Bad fats are found in margarine, shortening, baked goods, fast food and most restaurant fried foods.

If you're trying to avoid cholesterol, go for vegetable-based dishes. Note also that there is currently debate as to the difference between cholesterol in food and the cholesterol produced by the liver. While you wait for those-in-the-know to enlighten you, be sensible rather than jumping into a vat of ice cream.

Please do not be afraid of salad dressing, by which I mean vinaigrette with quality olive oil. You need the oil to help absorb the vitamins and minerals in the vegetables. In the words of Walter Willett, head of Harvard School of Public Health, "Eat your salad dressing but ditch the bread basket."

Speaking of bread, let's segue into the third macronutrient category: carbohydrates.

Carbs have been vilified with the advent of high-protein diets to the extent that some people are terrified to touch them. That's a shame. Carbohydrates in their natural format—fruit, vegetables and whole grains—are terrific foods, full of nutrients and fiber.

The problem occurs when carbs are stripped of their nutrients and "refined," ridding them of fiber and leaving a higher sugar content behind. Sugar is the root of all evil because it is highly acidic, very addictive and has profound effects on energy and mood. Excess sugar is stored in the body as fat. Next time you reach for a low-fat cookie, take heed that the fat doesn't make you fat, but the sugar does.

Look for good carbs in whole grains like brown rice, quinoa, barley, couscous and whole-wheat pasta. While some fruits contain high quantities of fructose, these are mitigated by the fiber and water content. Fruit grows on trees, so we're meant to eat it. The only problem is that we don't eat fruit seasonally any more, so it's all too easy for us to eat too much fruit that's very high in sugar, like mangoes and watermelon. Avoid fruit juices, as these have sky-high sugar contents, and take your time to munch through each piece of whole fruit so you benefit from the fiber.

By keeping good carbs in your diet, you'll find it easier to keep on an even keel energetically, and avoid digestive issues, especially when traveling.

Micronutrients are found in the body in minuscule amounts and are vital for the optimal function of most organ systems. Very small amounts are needed, but they choreograph a finely tuned dance that keeps us going and feeling good. In addition to overall well-being, micronutrients come into play seriously when we talk about jet lag and preventing illness.

You can get micronutrients from a varied diet of quality protein, fruit and vegetables, but they also come in a bottle and the booming supplement industry hopes you'll choose the latter. The argument is that as our food sources deteriorate (poor soil, genetically modified crops, pesticides), we don't derive the naturally occurring micronutrients we need from our diet. Hence the "need" for supplementation.

BEFORE CHANGING YOUR DIET, CHANGE YOUR MIND

I like to say there's so much more to eating than food. There are certain behavioral patterns that can affect digestion, how much you eat and how you feel after eating. These patterns include a few bad habits that travelers tend to display. You find yourself on the run, eating in your car, at your desk, in front of a screen, be it computer or TV. I think back to times I've ordered room service and stayed in my hotel room all evening doing paperwork and keeping half an eye on CNN. Before I knew it, everything on the tray would have disappeared.

Eating while distracted leads to eating about 30-percent more than you normally would (read Brian Wansink's awesome book *Mindless Eating: Why We Eat More Than We Think* for some interesting and fun tips on the topic). When you're distracted, your brain and belly are less likely to register that you're full. You're far more likely to stop eating only when the packet or plate is empty, or at the end of the program you're watching.

As for eating on the run, did you know that it takes 20 minutes after a meal for the brain and body to make the connection that you're full? This is why eating on the run leads to higher than normal consumption and indigestion. When you eat in what is essentially a distressed state, the digestive system acknowledges a condition of "fight or flight," making it harder to process food and absorb nutrients from it.

Unless you're working in a Mediterranean country, you're not going to have a two-hour lunch break. You have to find ways to take time out and give your meal the attention it deserves. Chewing your food thoroughly and putting your knife and fork down between bites helps. These behavioral components of digestion help the diminished parasympathetic control of digestion during stress. If you're in your car, park and get out. If you're in an office, move away from your desk to enjoy your meal. If it's available to you, go outside to eat, weather permitting. Anything to break up the overeating routine.

Another habit is one to which I've already confessed, that of purchasing a latte and chocolate cookies every time I went through an airport. I was following a pattern and all too frequently I see similar patterns with clients.

The key is to create new habits gradually without letting your brain think it is missing out. For example, my client Jim used to fly regularly from London to Athens. On his way through Terminal 3, he would stop at the pub for two pints of beer and a meat pie. We didn't want Jim to think he was missing out on his beer, so he started by having a glass of water with each pint, which meant he was able to cut down to two halves. Then he worked on replacing the meat pie with a healthier menu choice. Eventually he was able to cut out the habit all together (and save a few bucks!).

Another factor that affects eating habits is sleep patterns. When you don't have enough sleep, you wake up groggy and likely find yourself reaching for fatty, sugary foods for a quick jolt of energy. Smart choices come harder when you're tired, making you more likely to throw in the towel and mutter something about starting a healthy regimen tomorrow.

CHAPTER 2

WHY FREQUENT TRAVELERS REALLY NEED TO EXERCISE

When you hit the road, the road hits back. Hard.

Picture a typical day in the life of a frequent traveler. You're squashed into an airplane seat that was designed for increased airline profit not your comfort, and definitely not your well-being. You have no room to move, but you have to work on your laptop. Nifty travel pillow or not, your neck muscles are tightening more and more.

As you nod off, your head begins bouncing around more than a Bobblehead's. You can't adjust your chair for optimal ergonomics or lumbar support, but you can adjust it to enhance the misery of the person seated behind you.

> "IT IS AS IF SOME EVIL ENGINEER DESIGNED A PROGRAM TO INFLICT MAXIMUM WEAR AND TEAR ON YOUR BODY. IN SHORT, CONSTANT TRAVELING HAS TURNED YOU INTO A BIO- MECHANICAL NIGHTMARE BY PLACING TREMENDOUS AMOUNTS OF TORQUE ON YOUR TRUNK AND MAJOR JOINTS."

You're dehydrated. You're always dehydrated. Always exhausted. You are repeatedly leaning over in awkward, unbalanced positions to pick up luggage and load it onto conveyor belts or into overhead compartments. You sling your computer bag onto the same shoulder every time. You walk long distances through enormous terminals in heels, platforms or other nonsupportive shoes. It is as if some evil engineer designed a program to inflict maximum wear and tear on your body.

In short, constant traveling has turned you into a bio-mechanical nightmare by placing tremendous amounts of torque on your trunk and major joints. Any one of these actions, individually repeated, would stress your vertebral column, but done in combination on a constant, near-daily basis, it is little wonder you are extremely susceptible to lower back pain and other issues related with spinal compression, as well as a condition called forward head posture (see page 47 for more on FHP).

I think we all know, if maybe not fully understand, that spinal and vertebral column health are critical to our overall well-being. Your central nervous system extends nerves from your brain into the spinal column from where they disseminate peripherally throughout your body. The vertebrae that protect the spinal cord are separated and cushioned by intervertebral discs. (Think of them as pillows that need to stay fluffed so that the vertebral bones don't touch each other and impinge the nerves that leave the spinal column through the vertebrae.) When the discs are crushed, the result is pain and restricted movement. Intervertebral discs also dehydrate throughout the day so that you are actually shorter at night when you go to sleep than when you awaken in the morning.

The repetitive motion of certain actions, like those mentioned above, can cause the disks to desiccate asymetrically, causing them to wear thin and possibly herniate.

Sustained and repetitive flexion can compromise the protective action of the back muscles, which normally contract automatically. What does that mean? The girdle of muscles that protects your core will become compromised if measures aren't taken to strengthen and balance their agonist and antagonist relationship on a regular basis.

You may not be aware of what's happening, but one day, you bend down to pick up your bag and feel a shooting pain in your lower back. (Think of the person who says they simply bent over to pick up a pencil and their back "went.") Insidious injury from imbalance in the agonist/antagonist muscle action happens slowly and silently in many cases, until suddenly you experience traumatic pain.

A study in the *European Spine Journal* reports: "Sitting by itself does not increase the risk of lower back pain. However, sitting for more than half a work day, in combination with whole body vibration and/or awkward postures, does increase the likelihood of having lower back pain and/or sciatica, and it is the combination of these risk factors which leads to the greatest increase in lower back pain."

You don't have to have a doctorate in physiology to know the truth of this. The description sounds like torture. Or traveling.

Who sits for more than half a work day being subjected to whole body vibration and/or awkward postures? You, the constant traveler. Helicopter pilots have the greatest incidence of whole body vibration, but airline passengers cramped into tiny seats, attempting to sleep at strange angles, and not being permitted to get up and move around if the seatbelt sign is on can tell you all about awkward postures.

Being glued to electronic devices and hauling heavy carry-ons can be a pain in the neck, literally. Good posture and ergonomics are hard enough for the desk worker to achieve, but try typing with someone sitting less than a couple of inches away on either side of you. Looking down at a screen, texting and cell phone use all promote excessive flexion in the cervical spine (neck).

The same issues with desiccation and compression in the lower back apply also to the more delicate cervical vertebrae. Aside from the pain itself, cervical spine damage may lead to tingling and/or numbness in the wrists and hands, not to mention excruciating headaches, temporomandibular disorders (TMJ), and myofascial pain syndrome.

Overuse of hand-held devices combined with being continuously slumped forward while working at a computer has led to increased incidences of forward head posture, or FHP. (I think of FHP as "turtle neck" syndrome.) More people have FHP than they realize. Do you sit up straight and hold your phone in front of you while you text? Or do you hunch your shoulders, rounding your back and collapsing your chest as you thrust as your head forward to look at the screen?

Forward head posture is serious and once you let it develop, it takes serious effort to correct. For every one inch that your neck cranes forward, it has to hold an extra 10 pounds of weight in addition to the 12-pound power ball otherwise known as your head.

When lower back and neck pain become chronic, your quality of life and career longevity come into play. If your job requires globe-trotting or even state-hopping, you need to be able to get yourself across the state or across the globe with relative comfort and ease. When back or neck issues start, you'll feel lousy and your job performance will be affected. You'll need to take time off for doctor/chiropractor/osteopath/acupuncture appointments. You'll have trouble getting out of bed in the

"HELICOPTER PILOTS HAVE THE GREATEST INCIDENCE OF WHOLE BODY VIBRATION, BUT AIRLINE PASSENGERS CRAMPED INTO TINY SEATS, ATTEMPTING TO SLEEP AT STRANGE ANGLES, AND NOT BEING PERMITTED TO GET UP AND MOVE AROUND IF THE SEATBELT SIGN IS ON CAN TELL YOU ALL ABOUT AWKWARD POSTURES."

morning with or without medications. You may have to endure epidural injections or even contemplate surgery. If you are unable to do your work in a timely way, at some point, you may be passed over for someone healthier who can get the job done sooner. Or you could ignore your symptoms and suffer in silence for a very long time.

It sounds terrible. It *is* terrible. So what's to be done?

Mile High and Healthy offers a multifaceted program to ward off injury and rejuvenate even the veteran with enough Sky Miles to get to Pluto. The first step is a targeted exercise regimen—and more important, one that you can take on the road.

> "*MILE HIGH AND HEALTHY* OFFERS A MULTI-FACETED PROGRAM TO WARD OFF INJURY AND REJUVENATE EVEN THE VETERAN WITH ENOUGH SKY MILES TO GET TO PLUTO. THE FIRST STEP IS A TARGETED EXERCISE REGIMEN— AND IMPORTANTLY, ONE THAT YOU CAN TAKE ON THE ROAD."

The right exercise program will help ensure that your exposure to these issues is minimized. What's more, spinal compression aside, there are a slew of other reasons why road warriors should be taking a preventative approach to health with functional exercise.

8 MORE REASONS
TO EXERCISE

1 // **EXERCISE IS ENERGIZING AND INVIGORATING.** The intervertebral disks need movement for nourishment, especially rotation (which, ironically, is one of the most painful movements when disks are injured). Feeling invigorated means you'll have more energy to tackle your day. You will exude this energy when you present yourself to others.

2 // **BUSINESS TRAVELERS NEED TO BE PHYSICALLY STRONG.** Even if you have the latest in spine-friendly rolling luggage, you're still going to have to pick it up at some point for placement in an overhead compartment or on a hotel room luggage rack. Then there's your computer bag and, Ladies, that kitchen sink lurking in your handbag. A weak core and spaghetti arms will simply not suffice.

3 // **STRONG BONES ARE DE RIGUEUR.** I speak from my own experience here, having been diagnosed with osteopenia at an early age. Sedentary lifestyle, poor diet and lack of vitamin D have resulted in the increase of bone density issues beyond the traditional populations of small-boned women. The disease is actually becoming more prevalent among males. The unfortunate fact about osteoporosis is that it's known as the silent disease because of its as-ymptomatic nature. You can't feel or see that you have weakened bones so it's really important to have regular bone density tests. A consistent, healthy diet and plenty of weight-bearing exercise make an enormous difference.

4 // YOU NEED TO HAVE A HEALTHY HEART. While lugging bags as you traipse through airports certainly constitutes exercise, you're also sitting for hours in planes, cars and meetings. Long periods of being sedentary interrupted by sporadic bursts of heavy lifting are a recipe for cardiac problems. Of course stress doesn't help either, leaving the business traveler a (literal) sitting duck for the deadly duo of heart attacks and strokes.

5 // YOU WANT YOUR BLOOD TO BE OXYGENATED SO CELLS ARE NOURISHED AND THE CARDIOVASCULAR SYSTEM IS STRENGTHENED. The flow of oxygenated blood to the cells is crucial for overall well-being. If we don't look after our-selves at a cellular level, there's not much hope for the sum of all those cells, which is otherwise known as our body.

6 // YOU WANT TO AVOID ILLNESS ON THE ROAD. Think of all the lovely germs you encounter as you share space on airplanes, sleep in hotel rooms that a stranger occupied the night before and drive a rental car that was cleaned in haste and not necessarily sanitized. Exercise promotes good circulation, which means that the cells and other factors of the immune system are able to move through the body and take care of business. Research is preliminary at this stage, but the overall consensus is that exercise promotes overall good health which is vital for a healthy immune system.

7 // YOU WANT TO BE A CLEAR THINKER WITH A SHARP MEMORY. Know how you feel sluggish when you've been sitting for a while? A good workout will recharge your mental batteries and keep you focused. The hippocampus, the brain's memory center, has been shown to shrink as a result of poorly regulated blood sugar levels. By building muscle, you can regulate glucose levels, which will help ward off said shrinkage. If you are the type who gets inspired when they work out, have a voice recorder handy so you can record those pearls of wisdom.

> "THINK OF ALL THE LOVELY GERMS YOU ENCOUNTER AS YOU SHARE SPACE ON AIRPLANES, SLEEP IN HOTEL ROOMS THAT A STRANGER OCCUPIED THE NIGHT BEFORE, AND DRIVE A RENTAL CAR THAT WAS CLEANED IN HASTE AND NOT NECESSARILY SANITIZED."

8 // YOU WANT THE SATISFACTION OF ACCOMPLISHMENT. There's nothing like a good workout to make you feel like you can conquer the world. And, let's face it, you really might have to.

Being armed with good intentions is fabulous, but making them happen is the hard part. If ever there were a group of people who have difficulty finding time to exercise, it would be frequent travelers. Late arrivals, early meetings, travel days and business dinners all conspire against even the most well-intentioned individual to make sure that excuses not to exercise prevail.

Fortunately, *Mile High and Healthy* has answers that make sure exercise—not excuses—prevails.

ESSENTIAL EXERCISE
CORE STRENGTHENING

Core strength is essential for everyone. We all should work on our abdominal and back muscles, which form a corset-like protective layer for the spine and internal organs. But core conditioning is doubly important for the business traveler who is pulling, pushing, sitting and often slumped in cramped spaces for hours at a time.

> "CORE CONDITIONING IS DOUBLY IMPORTANT FOR THE BUSINESS TRAVELER WHO IS PULLING, PUSHING, SITTING AND OFTEN SLUMPED IN CRAMPED SPACES FOR HOURS AT A TIME. . . .STRENGTHENING YOUR CORE DOESN'T HAVE TO BE A DRAMATIC ORDEAL."

I've practiced Pilates for nearly 20 years, and am now a teacher of teachers internationally, with multiple certifications. Pilates focuses on core strength in a way that few other disciplines do, so I've seen many of the benefits first hand.

Strengthening your core doesn't have to be a dramatic ordeal. Like the rest of your life, it's about working smarter, not harder. You can develop your "Powerhouse," as Joseph Pilates called the group of muscles comprising the core, in five to ten minutes a day. This small investment of time and effort will help protect your back from undue damage.

The effect of strengthening and lengthening the spine helps create space between the vertebrae, essentially fluffing and nourishing the pillow-like discs. This in turn helps prevent desiccation and nerve impingement that lead to the conditions described earlier.

The stronger the abdominal girdle, the better your spinal alignment will be, all the way up to the neck. Core strength also protects your internal organs, decreases bloating and improves posture, which, by the way, makes you look taller and slimmer.

The most effective core strengthening exercises include flexion, rotation and extension. In other words, you need to bend, twist and stretch the spinal muscles in order to remain flexible.

The best way to achieve core strength is to work one-on-one with a professional, either a personal trainer or Pilates instructor, so that you can appreciate correct form and learn a repertoire of exercises you can do in your hotel room. (Most studios and gyms have introductory offers, so take advantage of this and work with different trainers to find the best fit for you). Investing in a few one-on-one sessions will ensure you learn good form and save you from potential injury once you start exercising on your own.

Alternatively, look for travel-friendly, downloadable workouts with a core-strengthening component (see Chapter 3). Another option would be an app like Runtastic Six-Pack Abs. This free app with avatar trainers lets you choose from 10-day programs and gradually increase the intensity as you strive to build your very own washboard abs.

Whichever option you choose, remember that consistency is the key to change. A few minutes a day invested in core strength can help stave off years of back pain.

DEALING WITH FORWARD HEAD POSTURE

The next step is to correct forward head posture. Thankfully the neck has some super big muscles to protect it so you can work on strengthening them and countering the hyperflexion typical of FHP. Aligning the neck correctly will help alleviate headaches, too.

To see if you have or are developing forward head posture, stand with your back, heels and the back of your head against a wall, making sure you don't hyperextend your neck. Can you do this easily? Does your head want to lean away from the wall? If you have difficulty placing your head against the wall, chances are that you have forward head posture and you might want to consult a chiropractor. Additionally, there are simple exercises you can do to gradually remedy FHP, even in a hotel room.

Stand with your back, heels and the back of the head against a wall. If your head can't touch the wall, place a pillow behind it. Lower and tuck in your chin to avoid hyperextending your neck. Place your arms by your side, palms facing your legs. Now raise your arms until there's a 45-degree angle between your arms and legs. This is your starting position. Lift and lower your arms against the wall 10 times.

Now come back to the starting position, gliding your arms up the wall, and cover your ears with your palms. Glide your arms back down to the starting position. Do 10 reps. Next, climb an imaginary rope ladder, pulling down on the "ladder" for 10 reps. Repeat each of the three exercises twice more. Do the entire sequence twice a day, and you should start to see and feel a difference within a month.

Now you have the information to help relieve two major chronic conditions. But how to fit exercise into your insanely busy schedule? Let's see how you can introduce more exercise into your routine, even if you think you have absolutely no time available to do so.

CHAPTER 3

FINDING TIME
TO EXERCISE

You leave home at 6 a.m. to catch an early flight. At your destination, you go right into meetings. After work, you stop at your hotel to drop off your luggage. You go out for dinner with clients or colleagues. After dinner, you return to the hotel and crash. The next day you do it all over again. When are you supposed to find time to exercise?

REALLY EASY WAYS TO BRING (MORE) EXERCISE INTO YOUR ROUTINE

1 // MOVE MORE. If the thought of exercising gives you the shivers, it's time to trick your brain. Don't set your goal to run a triathlon within the next two weeks. Rather, think in terms of simply moving more. The kind of movement you do may be walking an extra block or two, or using the hotel staircases instead of elevators. If you are so inclined, it might take the form of dancing around your hotel room to your favorite tunes.

Whatever you choose to do, if it's more than you're currently doing, that's wonderful. You can build on that when it becomes part of your routine, when you don't have to think about it anymore because it's second nature.

2 // SET REASONABLE GOALS. As a Pilates studio owner, I've seen many newcomers become so enthralled with their first session that they vow to come every day. Imagine the client's surprise when I advise against it. The overdoer rarely lasts two weeks, if that. I suggest working out twice a week until you're comfortable with the schedule. At that point you can add another session and, once that has become a habit, continue adding sessions until you are exercising every day.

3 // TAKE ADVANTAGE OF DOWN TIME AT AIRPORTS. When you have a delay or a long layover, you can sit and work, or you can work out. Even if you have lots of catching up to do, allocate a portion of your airport down time to moving. Read on for information about a variety of airport workout options.

4 // SCHEDULE YOUR WORKOUT TIME LIKE YOU WOULD A BUSINESS APPOINTMENT. Exercise needs to be a habit, not a whim. If you're a reluctant exerciser or you think you don't have time to exercise, the easiest way to make it a habit is to schedule your workouts like you would any meeting. Even if you're not training with an instructor or going to an exercise class, treat your workouts as though you are paying for them. Hold yourself to these appointments and make them a priority.

5 // CHUNK IT DOWN. Do you apply an all-or-nothing approach to working out? If you don't have time to work out for 30 minutes or an hour, do you think you've blown your opportunity? If you only have 10 minutes to exercise, that's okay. Give yourself permission for a shorter workout—it's still a workout.

You can get a lot done in a small amount of time, and chances are that once you allow yourself to shift away from all-or-nothing extreme, you'll find other slots in your day to fit in shorter workouts. Before you know it, you'll be doing over 30 minutes a day without having to carve out larger chunks of time over fewer days.

6 // DO 10 MINUTES IF THAT'S ALL YOU CAN MANAGE. Ten minutes are better than no minutes. If all you have time for today is 10 minutes of ab work, that's enough time to lengthen your spine, so you'll be sitting up straight all day. You can strive to do more tomorrow.

7 // BE ACCOUNTABLE. There is nothing like an accountability partner to keep you true to yourself. Whether your partner is a trainer, an app, a colleague or a friend, you will be more likely to put in the effort if you know you have to answer to someone else besides yourself. Studies show that 95% of people who exercise with a partner stick with it, compared with 43% who work out alone (per exercisefriends.com 2013).

You don't have to work out together, just check in with each other. It can be as much or as little as a Tweet. You can also use a free app like Pump Up, which connects you with like-minded people as you work towards your fitness goals together.

8 // Use an app. Years ago, I used to travel with a list of exercises that I faithfully performed each day. How prehistoric compared with today when I can pull up Pilates Anytime on my phone and work out with a different teacher every day. New fitness apps are popping up all the time, and there's definitely something for everyone.

Popular free apps include FitStar Personal Trainer, Nike+ Training Club, Fitnet and Sworkit (designed specifically for busy people). You can also use apps to track your progress. Try Argus, MapMyFitness and Endomondo.

9 // Take advantage of connectivity. If you have a trainer and can keep working with them via Skype or FaceTime, please do. A creative and experienced trainer will be able to devise effective in-room workouts for you from 10 to 60 minutes long. You can keep your workouts going and progress accordingly. If you haven't tried virtual workouts, take a test session with someone that offers them to see if that modality can work for you.

10 // Pay in advance. Book a session with a trainer at your destination. Chances are you'll have to deal with a 24-hour cancellation policy so you'll be obliged to keep your session. The thought of losing money can be a great motivator. This won't work for those whose travel plans change frequently. You want to be in the same city as your trainer, unless you're working out via Skype, as suggested above.

WEARABLE DEVICES

In this day and age, your accountability partner may well be a wearable device. The use of watch-like items—that track how far you walk or jog or how long you sleep—is set to escalate at a compound annual rate of 35% over the next five years, reaching 148 million units shipped annually in 2019, up from 33 million units shipped in 2014, according to a 2015 report by *Business Insider*.

You can use the device to be accountable to yourself, or you can compete with family, friends and colleagues via an app or companion web account. Wearables provide a way to monitor your progress by tracking your activity as well as your weight, metrics and food intake. They typically sync to your phone or computer.

> "SCHEDULE YOUR WORKOUT TIME LIKE YOU WOULD A BUSINESS APPOINTMENT. EXERCISE NEEDS TO BE A HABIT, NOT A WHIM. IF YOU'RE A RELUCTANT EXERCISER OR YOU THINK YOU DON'T HAVE TIME TO EXERCISE, THE EASIEST WAY TO MAKE IT A HABIT IS TO SCHEDULE YOUR WORKOUTS LIKE YOU WOULD ANY MEETING."

Since wearables are updating faster than we can publish, check out pcmag.com for an updated comparison of the latest models. FitBit dominates the market with 67% share in 2013 (NPD Group Wearable Technology Report, Jan 2014) for its Fitbit Surge and Fitbit Charge HR. Other popular models are Garmin's Vivoactive and Vivosmart, the Basis Peak, Mio Fuse and the Jawbone UP24. Your choice will likely depend on desired bells and whistles as well as budget.

WHERE TO EXERCISE ON THE GO
HOTEL ROOM

If you prefer to work out in private, don't feel safe venturing outside or your hotel has a subpar workout facility, your room provides a wider variety of fitness options than you might think. If you don't have the luggage space to carry a mat with you and the hotel doesn't have loaners, fold up your bedspread to form a mat. You're now set for yoga, Pilates and ab and plank routines.

If you're into barre sequences, use the desk chair as an impromptu ballet barre. Speaking of bars, cans from the mini bar work great as light hand weights, unless it's one of those horrible contraptions that charge you every time you remove an item.

Typically, you'll be using your own body weight for resistance or small, lightweight portable props. The latter would include therabands, the Pilates Magic Circle, resistance tubes and gliding discs.

You can do your own routine, or follow an app or a Skype session as described above. Alternatively, download a workout to your laptop or tablet. For Pilates, try pilatesology.com to take advantage of a 10-day free trial with sessions from highly reputable teachers. For yoga, choose from yogadownload.com, gaiamtv.com (subscription service) and yogaglo.com (subscription service but also offers a 15-day free trial). Physique57. com offers a variety of barre workouts for individual purchase or by subscription.

YouTube.com has a slew of downloadable workouts for resistance bands and tubes. When you find a workout that appeals to you, be sure to check out the trainer's credentials because amateurs can post there too. You don't want to be writhing in pain on your hotel room floor because the unaccredited instructor overlooked safety precautions. (This is why Skype workouts are a really good idea for in-room practice).

As for cardio, I used to do jumping jacks and burpees in my hotel room, although I always worried about disturbing the folks in the room below me. Then I discovered gliding discs. Although I've been told that you can just as easily use paper plates, I highly recommend buying the real deal at gliding-discs.com so you have the accompanying DVD. Gliding disc workouts will raise your heart rate without having to set foot outside your hotel room. They are perfect for as brief as a five-minute cardio session when you're pressed for time. Best of all, they weigh practically nothing and easily fit into hand luggage.

Finally, a word of caution thanks to a CEO I know. Being the creative type, he decided to do pull-ups using the doorjamb of his hotel room in an older London property. You guessed it, the whole thing pulled out of the wall and came crashing down. Try explaining that one to housekeeping.

HOTEL GYM

Not all hotel workout rooms are created equal. Some are spectacular. Many are afterthoughts. Dark, dank holes at the end of long corridors send me scurrying back to my room to practice Pilates. The Rosewood Crescent in Dallas and the Waldorf Astoria Spa at El Conquistador in Puerto Rico have me strutting my stuff. The truth is, world-class spa or dingy dive—both get the job done. Walking through the door will always be the most important step.

If you prefer to use the hotel gym, make sure that whoever is booking your travel knows that this is a priority for you. My recommendations are:

EVEN HOTELS

IHG launched an entire brand around health conscious travel in 2014. EVEN Hotels properties boast well-appointed and spacious gyms called Athletic Studios with plenty of the latest equipment, plus a separate room for yoga and stretching ("Flex Room").

If you prefer company while you work out, staff members jump in daily to lead classes and activities on property and off. Prefer privacy? Rooms have dedicated workout spaces with cork flooring and a mounted fitness wall. A yoga mat and props, exercise ball and resistance bands are provided. If you don't have your own routine, you can take advantage of the in-room exercise manual and 19 TV channels with guided workouts.

WESTIN HOTELS & RESORTS

WestinWORKOUT rooms are offered at participating properties, giving you the choice of an in-room treadmill or stationary bike. You can also request dumbbells, fitness DVDs, resistance bands and stability balls. If jogging is your thing, the Run-WESTIN™ program helps you select between 3- and 5-mile trails, possibly with a running concierge. Otherwise you'll be provided with trail maps. WestinWORKOUT Workout Fitness Centers are on the better end of the hotel gym scale. Plus, for

$5 you can rent New Balance shoes and clothing, meaning sneakers don't have to take up half of your carry-on.

EQUINOX

The folks at Equinox have taken their leading gym brand and created a hotel around it. And not just any old gym, the first Equinox Hotel will be home to the world's largest Equinox fitness center at 60,000 square feet. The New York City property will open in 2018, followed by LA in 2019, continuing until Equinox reaches its target of 75 hotels worldwide.

> "NOT ALL HOTEL WORK-OUT ROOMS ARE CREATED EQUAL. SOME ARE SPECTACULAR. MANY ARE AFTERTHOUGHTS. DARK, DANK HOLES AT THE END OF LONG CORRIDORS SEND ME SCURRYING TO MY ROOM TO PRACTICE PILATES."

HOTEL POOL

Swimming is great full-body exercise, and what can be easier than simply having to pack a swimsuit? As long as the water temperature's right, squeezing in some early morning or evening laps is an effective way to combat stress and stretch your body at the same time. Swimming should never be your only exercise, because it isn't weight-bearing and won't help you build bone density, but it's a valuable component of an overall fitness regime.

OUTSIDE GYM

If your hotel doesn't have a gym, you may well be able to find one nearby. Disappointment in an LA hotel's workout room was rapidly assuaged when I spotted an LA Fitness across the street. Suddenly, there was the opportunity to take a variety of classes and work with a trainer. Access to a full facility and trainers enables you to vary your workouts and keep them interesting, while respecting form and safety.

> "YOU CAN FINALLY WAVE GOODBYE TO THE NOISY BAR, TACKLING PAPERWORK OR OTHER UNAPPEALING OPTIONS WHILE YOU WAIT. WITH THE *MILE HIGH AND HEALTHY* MENTALITY, AIRPORTS CAN BECOME A GREAT PLACE TO EXERCISE."

PILATES OR YOGA STUDIO

If you're a yoga, barre or Pilates fan, find a studio near your location and book sessions in advance of your trip so you have no excuses. Most studios will require payment in advance, or they'll have a 24-hour cancelation policy. That's a real incentive! Mindbodyonline.com is a good resource for finding studios.

GET OUTSIDE

Business travelers are indoor creatures. You're in planes, offices, rental cars, taxis, airports and, quite often, restaurants. Yet, exposure to the great outdoors is one of the most rewarding gifts you can give yourself. Exposure to natural light has a positive effect on your circadian rhythms, which helps with jet lag, is a source of vitamin D, aids in stress release, eases brain fog and contributes overall feelings of well-being.

Many joggers swear by maintaining their routine while they are traveling, and some hotels are doing their bit with dedicated jogging paths/running trails on property or simply offering maps showing local trails. Jogging also allows travelers the opportunity to explore a new urban neighborhood, or even wilder terrain.

That said, the newness of the surroundings may in itself pose an issue, depending on the city or the country. Female travelers especially may feel less inclined to maintain a jogging or walking schedule if they don't feel safe. Packs of dogs in Africa and even on certain Caribbean beaches have thwarted many of my attempts to explore a new destination à pied. Check with the hotel concierge if you'd like to avoid surprises.

Check out the free app Spring, which plays songs with a similar range of beats per minute so you can run along to them. Just don't wear leg warmers and a headband.

AT THE AIRPORT

There's somewhat of a revolution taking place right now. Many airports are going to great lengths to keep waiting passengers happy, and this includes fitness.

You can finally wave goodbye to the noisy bar, tackling paperwork or other unappealing options while you wait. With the *Mile High and Healthy* mentality, airports can become a great place to exercise. Depending on your location, you may be golfing, bicycling, swimming, inline skating or practicing yoga.

AIRPORT GYMS

The horizon for airport gyms is looking extremely bright with the launch of AirFit, which is bringing dedicated, fully equipped gym facilities to post-security retail spaces in airports throughout the US. With strong interest from JFK and SFO to start, expect to see AirFit expand to most major US airports over the next few years. Check airfit.us for updates.

If you're looking for an airport gym, the big question is going to be whether or not you're willing to go off property during your layover. Airportgyms.com lists fitness facilities that are on site and within proximity of US and Canadian airports.

While it's a great idea to work out before you fly, there's the issue of personal hygiene and whether or not you'd like to stuff your sweaty workout clothes in your hand luggage. Locations with showers and laundry facilities are the most practical. If laundry isn't on your airport time to-do list, I strongly suggest investing in something a little sturdier than a Ziploc to store your sweaty clothes until you reach your destination. Try The Sweaty Bag (omeomyproducts.com) or The Sweat Mate (the-sweatmate.com).

Here are my top 10 recommendations for airport gyms. (Hours and prices were accurate when this book went to press, but are subject to change.)

1 // SINGAPORE CHANGI AIRPORT'S AMBASSADOR TRANSIT LOUNGE at Terminal 2 is open 24 hours a day. And since it is in a transit lounge, it is located airside. For just S$26, you can work out in the fully equipped gym, rent workout clothes and take a shower with basic toiletries provided. If you bring your own togs, it's S$17.

2 // TORONTO PEARSON INTERNATIONAL AIRPORT has a state-of-the-art gym concession courtesy of Goodlife Fitness, Canada's largest fitness company. Located pre-security in the Terminal 1 arrivals Area F, the facility is open from 4 a.m. to 11:30 p.m. The daily fee is C$15 per person, while current GoodLife members may be able to use it for free, depending on their membership level. You can rent a Reebok clothing and shoe bundle for C$10. Luggage storage, towel service and showers with amenities are all at your disposal.

3 // VANCOUVER INTERNATIONAL AIRPORT's 24-hour gym is located on the lobby level of the Fairmont Hotel right inside the terminal, above US check-in. The Health Club boasts a gym, saunas, whirlpool and three-lane lap pool. It's open 6:30 a.m. to 11 p.m. for hotel guests and drop-in visitors and 24-hours a day for Fairmont Gold and Fairmont Presidents Club members. Drop-ins pay C$18 per visit for access to the Health Club, saunas and showers. Shorts, sneakers and a shirt can be rented for C$10.

4 // LONDON HEATHROW AIRPORT has two onsite gyms, one at the Hilton located within Terminal 4 and one at the Sofitel at Terminal 5, accessible by a bridge. The Hilton facility is operated by the LivingWell chain and sports Precor equipment, an indoor pool, showers and a team of personal trainers.

A day pass for the club is £20 or £10 if you are a Hilton Honours member. If you know ahead of time that you'll be there, visit payasugym.com to purchase a day pass for the discounted price of £8.75. LivingWell Heathrow is open Monday to Friday from 6 a.m. to 10 p.m. and Saturday and Sunday from 8 a.m. to 9 p.m. The Sofitel's pool, sauna, spa and fitness center can be accessed for a £25 fee if a spa treatment isn't booked or you're not a hotel resident. This impressive facility is open 24 hours.

5 // AMSTERDAM'S SCHIPHOL AIRPORT offers a host of activities, not least a top-notch 24-hour gym and spa at the Sheraton

Amsterdam Airport Hotel, which is located between Schiphol Plaza and the World Trade Center. Day passes are offered for €20 or €27.50 which includes a food and beverage voucher for the Runway Café. With a day pass, you can use the fitness center, sauna, rainforest showers, steam room and the wellness area.

6 // THE HILTON CHICAGO O'HARE AIRPORT is connected to domestic terminals by underground walkways. Terminal 5 passengers can take a complimentary shuttle. You can purchase a day pass for $20 ($22.40 with tax) and use the Fitness Center, indoor Olympic size pool, sauna, steam room and showers. Hours are 5 a.m. to 10 p.m. on weekdays, 6 a.m. to 10 p.m. on weekends.

7 // THE WESTIN DETROIT METROPOLITAN AIRPORT HOTEL is connected to the World Gateway Terminal and a complimentary 24-hour shuttle to the North Terminal. The property features the signature WestinWorkout Fitness Studio® which nonguests can use for $15 a day. While Westin was one of the first hotels to rent workout clothes, be aware that this service is for hotel guests only.

8 // DUBAI is a major gateway to the Middle and Far East and thus a stopover for many passengers. Thankfully, this airport sports one of the fanciest onsite health clubs, with locations in Concourses B and C. In addition to the 24-hour gym, which is available to use for $13 an hour, there are private showers plus men's and women's steam rooms, saunas and Jacuzzis to provide the opportunity to relax while waiting for your next flight. Swedish and shiatsu massages are also available.

9 // DALLAS FORT WORTH—meet the Grand Hyatt DFW at Terminal D, accessible by SkyLink and Terminal Link from other terminals. The skySPA offers a $30 day pass for access to the fitness center, outdoor saline pools, steam rooms and showers. Hours for passes are 9 a.m.to 5 p.m.

10 // THE HILTON MUNICH AIRPORT is within walking distance of Terminals 1 and 2. The 24-hour air-conditioned gym is fully equipped and there's a 17-meter long pool. Purchase a two-hour pass for €20 or a day pass for €30 and enjoy the Jacuzzi, solarium, sauna, steam bath, plus a towel and bathrobe to boot. The fitness center is open 24 hours, while the spa's hours are 7 a.m.to 10 p.m. Monday to Friday, and 8 a.m. to 10 p.m. weekends.

AIRPORT WALKING PATHS

Airport terminals are like mini climate-controlled tracks providing the perfect spot for a stroll without sweating profusely or freezing your socks off. You've probably trekked through airports without even realizing how much distance you were clocking. (If you've been through Miami, Frankfurt or Madrid, you know what I mean). While moving walkways are there to make things easier for you, make it easier to stay fit by ignoring them and using your legs.

The American Council on Sports Medicine has formed a task

force on healthy air travel and is working with airports to help them explore ways to provide healthier opportunities for passengers. You'll find quite a few dedicated walking paths in terminals so you can work towards your 10,000 steps before departure. Be warned that most airport websites aren't exactly promoting the fact that they have walking paths. They apparently want you to shop and eat while you wait. Check the list below to see if your frequent pit stop fits the bill. If not, forge your own path. But before you charge off in the name of health, as with any kind of exercise, form is key.

If you're walking the concourse and you have to take luggage with you, be mindful of your posture as you do so. Your hips and shoulders should be in line with each other, forming a "box" so that one shoulder isn't being pulled behind by your luggage. Make sure your lower back isn't arching. If it is, chances are your abs are slack and your core muscles aren't protecting your lower back. Curl your tailbone under slightly to counter the arch and soften the knees. Draw the abs in and up, and you're ready to go.

//HANDY HINT//

If you don't want to travel in sneakers or lug them with you, try Sketchers Go Walk line. They look better than sneakers if you're wearing business clothes, but you can also fold them up and stick them in your hand luggage. They're flexible and weigh practically nothing.

MOST AWESOME AIRPORT WALKING PATHS

1 // ANCHORAGE INTERNATIONAL AIRPORT has a 4.2-mile paved trail around the Lake Hood Seaplane Base. Baggage storage is available.

2 // HARTSFIELD-JACKSON ATLANTA INTERNATIONAL AIRPORT has a 7.9-mile walking path between terminals A and E.

3 // BALTIMORE-WASHINGTON INTERNATIONAL has a 12.5-mile paved trail, park including playground and an observation area for watching planes, all outside.

4 // BOSTON LOGAN has walking paths, health stations to check blood pressure, BMI (body mass index), height and weight.

5 // CLEVELAND HOPKINS INTERNATIONAL AIRPORT has the CLE Health Walk, a two-mile trek.

6 // DALLAS FORT WORTH has the LiveWell Walking Path, .7 miles in Terminal D, from gate D6 to D40. There are two step courses and a 55-foot high staircases at both Skylink Mover stations.

7 // FORT LAUDERDALE – HOLLYWOOD INTERNATIONAL AIRPORT has an outside, 1.3-mile Fit-Walking Path between terminals. There's a concession for bag storage.

8 // INDIANAPOLIS INTERNATIONAL AIRPORT has three walking paths: a quarter mile stretch in the ticket hall, plus a half mile and a 1.1- mile track around both concourses post-security.

9 // MINNEAPOLIS ST. PAUL AIRPORT has a post-security quarter mile track. Secure lockers are available to store your stuff.

10 // NEW ORLEANS has a half-mile course, but it is outside the secure area.

11 // PHOENIX SKY HARBOR has a two-mile post-security PHX Fitness Trail around Terminal 4, with seven free bottle-filling water stations. Baggage storage is not offered.

12 // SAN DIEGO INTERNATIONAL AIRPORT has a path for bicycles and pedestrians to points in the city

13 // SEATTLE TACOMA offers a two-mile stroll if you walk between Concourses A, B, C and D.

AIRPORT YOGA STUDIOS

Yoga studios are popping up at airports at about the same rate as food trucks, which means not fast enough. Hopefully, we'll see the trend increase, both within the US and abroad. Here's what's out there so far.

★ Dallas-Fort Worth International Airport has a dedicated yoga studio located after security by Gate D 40 in the hallway connecting terminals B&D. Use of the room is free of charge and mats are provided. The yoga room is open 24-hours a day, seven days a week.

★ San Francisco International Airport boasts two yoga rooms, both open 24-hours daily and post-security, one at Terminal 2 between Terminal 1, boarding area C and Terminal 2, boarding area D. The other is at Terminal 3, boarding area E, near gate 69. Mats and a variety of props are provided.

★ Burlington International Airport's yoga room is sponsored by a local studio, and so is well equipped with mats and props. Located before security, the studio is open from 4 a.m. until 10 p.m.

★ Chicago O'Hare International Airport's yoga studio is open from 6 a.m. to 10 p.m. daily. Mats are provided. The studio is located in Terminal 3, adjacent to the indoor urban garden on the mezzanine level of the rotunda.

★ Chicago Midway's yoga room has yoga mats, mirrors and there's no charge for use. Located airside in C concourse, the room is open from 6 a.m. to 10 p.m.

★ Helsinki Airport, Finland, offers an entire facility devoted to pre-flight relaxation. The 24-hour Kainuu lounge is located at gate 31 and mats are provided. You can also relax on ergonomic chairs and pick up reading material at the book swap.

★ London Heathrow's Terminal 4 yoga facility is unfortunately not open to all passengers as it's in the SkyTeam Lounge (opposite gate 10), but if you're not a member, you can purchase a day pass for £27.50, which includes all this plush lounge's facilities, including day beds, wellness center and showers. Mats are provided.

If walking the terminal is too pedestrian for you (couldn't resist), there are more extraordinary airport activities to be found around the world. Heading to Seoul, Korea? Check out Incheon International Airport's ice skating rink. Rent a stationary recharging bike at Amsterdam's Schipol Airport and charge your phone while you work out. Munich Airport offers 18 holes of mini golf at its Visitors Park, which is a three-minute shuttle ride from the airport. If you want the real thing, Hong Kong International boasts the Sky City Nine Eagles Golf Course, the city's first nine-hole course set to United States Golf Association standards.

Take all of this into account and you're going to be hoping for a long layover.

CHAPTER 4

FUELING
FOR ENERGY

Energy lulls are the bane of the frequent traveler. It isn't easy to sit in an office for 10 hours a day, but there's nothing like having to constantly be on the go. You're always moving from home to hotel to office, always having to be "on" and contend with surprises. You wake up in one city or country and go to sleep in another, sometimes several times a week.

I used to dash through airports grabbing lattes and chocolate graham cookies to "fuel" me through my trip. I was basically eating sugar on sugar on sugar with some caffeine thrown into the mix! Shock Alert: I had trouble sleeping at night.

So I spent half the day exhausted, trying to operate at about

50 percent. When I needed turbo fuel, I'd reach for caffeine. Again, unable to go to sleep at night, I'd have a glass of wine to help. This is not a healthy cycle, to say the least. How can it be broken?

Gaining more energy is pretty straightforward. It's all about what you consume. Energy is produced by dynamic factories in the cells called mitochondria. Glucose is the primary fuel mitochondria need to start the process. Glucose is the simplest form of carbohydrates. Dietary fats, as well as proteins, can make their way into the mitochondria as well, but glucose is the first to go.

> "THE REFINED OR "WHITE" CARBS THAT ARE READILY AVAILABLE AT AIRPORT FAST FOOD JOINTS SEND GLUCOSE TO THE BLOOD STREAM ON BIOLOGICAL HIGH SPEED TRAINS. CELLS ABSORB THE GLUCOSE SUPER FAST AND YOUR BLOOD SUGAR DROPS. IT'S TIME TO EAT AGAIN. BUT WAIT, YOU HAD THAT CINNAMON ROLL AN HOUR AGO. YOU ARE NOW OFFICIALLY ON AN ENERGY ROLLER COASTER."

Let's say you're feeling tired and peckish, so you pick up a cinnamon roll at the airport. What happens?

Sugar hits your mouth and starts getting digested right away. The liver gives a shout to the pancreas to release some insulin, which is a signal to the cells to absorb the blood sugar so that the mitochondria can produce energy. One long production chain is in motion. The sugar (now glucose) in the blood is gradually absorbed by the cells and blood sugar levels drop. It's time to eat and refuel.

The frequency with which you need to refuel depends on how fast the food you have consumed releases glucose. The refined or "white" carbs that are readily available at airport fast food concessions send glucose to the blood stream on biological high-speed trains. Cells absorb the glucose super fast, and your blood sugar drops. It's time to eat again. But wait, you had that cinnamon roll an hour ago. You are now officially on an energy roller coaster.

You start to feel tired and grumpy, maybe a little foggy. Twenty-five percent of the glucose you consumed went to your brain and central nervous system because they need it to function effectively, and now there's none left. So, you grab a slice of pizza and the whole process starts over. You experience another slump mid-afternoon, so you grab a coffee and a couple of cookies. Repeat.

Now you've eaten again so you should be feeling better, but that brain fog is still there. If the brain and central nervous system need carbohydrates to function, what's going wrong?

The refined carbs that you're consuming usually don't contain any fiber, so they go through the whole production line process really quickly. When carbs are whole grains they contain fiber, which slows down the production line.

The Glycemic Index (GI) is a measure of how blood sugar levels rise after eating different carbohydrates, with glucose having an index of 100. A banana is indexed at 62, black beans are 30, and carrots are 35. The speed with which blood sugar rises is affected by fat, protein and other nutrients in food, but only carbs are measured for the GI.

The glycemic index is not always the best measure for selecting a food, meaning you have to use smarts with it sometimes. For example, a Snickers bar has a glycemic index of 68 while a sweet potato is 70. Obviously, the sweet potato is more nutritionally dense.

A related measure is the glycemic load (GL), in which the glycemic index is multiplied by the net number of carbs in an actual serving of food. Even though the sweet potato has a relatively high GI, you would have to eat a large serving to cause the same insulin surge as the Snickers bar. The sweet potato's GL is 22 for an average size spud, whereas the Snickers is 46 for the whole bar.

The lower glycemic load is important for travelers because you want a slow release of glucose into the bloodstream so you stay full longer, concentrate better and avoid energy highs and lows. Some of the glucose turns into glycogen for storage in the liver, which releases it as needed. Your energy production line keeps going for as long as 12 hours, or as long as the glycogen supply in the liver will last.

You can step off the energy roller coaster at any time. You can do a double somersault, land on your feet and wave to everyone as they go rolling by. It's really that simple. Here's how.

"THE GLYCEMIC INDEX IS NOT ALWAYS THE BEST MEASURE FOR SELECTING A FOOD, MEANING YOU HAVE TO USE SMARTS WITH IT SOMETIMES. FOR EXAMPLE, A SNICKERS BAR HAS A GLYCEMIC INDEX OF 68 WHILE A SWEET POTATO IS 70. OBVIOUSLY THE SWEET POTATO IS MORE NUTRITIONALLY DENSE."

FIVE WAYS
TO AVOID SUGAR SURGES AND HAVE MORE ENERGY

1 // DITCH REFINED "WHITE" CARBS.

Instead, opt for whole grains and fiber, which slows the release of glucose (sugar) into your bloodstream. Slow and easy means sugar doesn't go from the blood into the cells as quickly, leaving your blood sugar steady for longer.

Switch white bread, pasta and rice for whole grains. Fruit and vegetables are also rich in fiber, so try to include them with every meal. Beans are best, as they break down slowly and release glucose gradually. Legume is the collective name for beans, lentils and chickpeas. They have ridiculous amounts of fiber, which is why I eat them in some form every day. Legumes aren't that hard to find on the road. Look for bean soups such as pasta e fagioli or lentil, hummus or white bean dips, and lentil or chickpea salad.

2 // EAT FAT AND PROTEIN WITH YOUR CARBOHYDRATES.

These other two macronutrients can also be used by the body to build sugar molecules, but the process takes several hours, compared with just minutes for carbs. Having a good mix of the three major nutrients slows down the release of sugar into the bloodstream and steers you away from the energy roller coaster.

Ideally you would opt for a fibrous carb, but sometimes life happens and your only option is regular pasta or white bread. To avoid the need for an afternoon nap, have veggies (red sauce counts) and meat or seafood with pasta or a sandwich with lean protein and veggies (cram as much lettuce, tomato and cucumber as you can on it) or a bean burrito with guacamole.

3 // CHOOSE THE RIGHT BREAKFAST.

To avoid initiating the energy roller coaster, begin with breakfast. Hidden sugar abounds in baked goods, cereals, juices, jams and jellies. Even the milk you might use in coffee or tea contains sugar. You add up all of that for a standard continental breakfast, and you're on the road to a mid-morning crash and burn. Hotels tend to offer continental breakfasts for free because they're cheap. They're also a blood sugar disaster.

> "HOTELS TEND TO OFFER CONTINENTAL BREAKFASTS FOR FREE BECAUSE THEY'RE CHEAP. THEY'RE ALSO A BLOOD SUGAR DISASTER. . . . SOMETIMES YOU HAVE TO BE A PAIN AND ASK FOR WHAT YOU WANT."

If continental is your only option, look for whole wheat bread, top with a little butter and just a teaspoon rather than a ladle of jam. Pick oatmeal rather than a sugary cereal. If you can get berries and nuts with it, even better. Fill up with fresh fruit and plain yogurt. I travel with a bag of chopped almonds and dried berries to tart up oatmeal and yogurt. They serve as a Scooby snack, too, in a pinch.

In a full-service establishment, you stand more chance of finding the perfect combo of fat, fiber and protein. Go for an omelet with lots of veggies and a sprinkling of cheese or lean meat with sautéed mushrooms, spinach, grilled tomatoes or any other veggies available. Huevos rancheros will do the trick, as will eggs Florentine on a whole wheat muffin, just use a light touch with the sauce. Avoid the accompanying breadbasket and mountain of home fries.

Repeat: Avoid the accompanying breadbasket and mountain of home fries.

Sometimes you have to be a pain and ask for what you want. My current breakfast of choice is whole wheat toast topped with mashed avocado and a squeeze of lemon. Or, I'll ask for sautéed spinach and onions with a poached or fried egg on top. It's not on the menu, but most restaurants can rustle up spinach and onion.

If you're having oatmeal or a high-fiber cereal, ask for unsweetened almond milk. Even if it's not available, the more you ask, the more the hotel will get the idea and perhaps make more options available for health conscious travelers in the future. I'm not averse to calling ahead and requesting what I want. I mean, we're talking self-described FULL- service establishments here.

4 // KEEP HEALTHY SNACKS ON HAND.

Many people use snacks to tide them over until their next meal. Road warriors sometimes end up having snacks instead of a meal! Unfortunately, most prepackaged snacks have hidden and not-so-hidden sugars. You have to be a sleuth to find the fat, fiber and protein combo.

Nuts are a great choice as long as they're portion controlled, like the mini-packs of pistachios you'll find at the supermarket. I take baggies of almonds, goji berries and raw chocolate nibs with me, or I make a batch of tamari almonds before a trip. (Heat tamari in a small skillet, add almonds and stir until nuts have absorbed the tamari, cook 1 minute longer, cool and bag).

Tubs of hummus and salsa with organic chips are good for a flight (I portion out Late July's organic chips). Try natural popcorn without artificial flavorings, such as Trader Joe's Organic Popcorn with Olive Oil. Be sure to portion it into baggies, or you'll eat the whole lot. Or at least, I will.

Seaweed snacks are fabulous. These are little sheets of roasted nori that come in small packages and are obviously very light to carry. Just check your teeth for green bits afterwards unless you want to look really silly.

> "A BADLY COMBINED MEAL WILL TAKE UP TO 40 HOURS TO TAKE THAT LITTLE JOURNEY, USING A TREMENDOUS AMOUNT OF ENERGY ALONG THE WAY."

5 // COMBINE YOUR FOODS WISELY.

When you eat a big dinner, the body can produce a flood of insulin. Consequently, many nutrition experts recommend eating smaller meals throughout the day. There are two problems with that. For one thing, some people don't like to eat that often. For another, it's completely impractical for anyone trying to get business done. "Hang on, I need to have another meal!" won't go down well in the middle of an interview or meeting.

Nine times out of ten you're going to be stuck with the big, protein-heavy meal at night, which is much harder and takes much longer to digest. You may find yourself lying in bed wondering if you're ever going to sleep. The next day, you are tired and lethargic.

One way to have more energy is to tax the digestive system less. The body uses between 5 and 15% of ingested calories to digest food. In fact, digestion is the most energy-consuming function of the body. It must be done right, or you won't assimilate nutrients from your food intake.

Food combining is based on the concept that the simpler the meal, the easier it is to digest. The most basic principle involves not mixing proteins and starches. So, meat or fish wouldn't combine with rice or starchy veggies such as potatoes or breads, the reason being these combinations linger in the digestive system for many hours, working their way out of the stomach then down 30 feet or so of intestinal tract.

A badly combined meal will take up to 40 hours to take that little journey, using a tremendous amount of energy along the way.

By contrast, having meat or fish with vegetables or salad, or pairing pasta with vegetables or a marinara sauce, means that the meal is digested more quickly and easily; you expend less energy on digestion, saving it for physical activity or brain power; and you won't want to take a nap after each meal. The faster a food passes through your system, providing you with adequate nutrition and then exiting, the healthier it is.

FOOD COMBINING CHEAT SHEET

1 // Proteins and starches do not mix. No meat sandwiches. No pasta and meatballs. No California rolls. Cheeseburgers and fries? Bagels and cream cheese? Do you even need to ask?

2 // Proteins do mix with vegetables. Have a salad to start your meal, then meat or fish with veggies. Grilled fish on a bed of greens? Superb. Steak sautéed with spinach—yep.

3 // Starches do mix with vegetables. That's vegetable risottos, pasta primavera, baked sweet potato and salad.

4 // Different starches do mix. That's rice and beans or black bean tacos or even a bean burrito.

5 // Different proteins do not mix. Protein is the hardest type of food to digest. The simpler you can keep it, the better. That means digesting one protein at a time. A fish appetizer followed by, say, a beef or pork main course won't work. But fish followed by fish or poultry followed by poultry will work.

6 // Fats do not mix well with protein—pair moderately. A little salad dressing is fine. Cheese on your burger isn't.

7 // Fats do mix with starches. That's license for pasta with oil and garlic or pumpkin or mushroom ravioli with sage butter sauce. It also means you can put a little butter on a baked sweet potato or add guacamole or hummus with chips or veggies. Avocado sushi rolls fit the bill, too.

8 // Fruits should be eaten on an empty stomach. There's a reason for this. Fruit has to be allowed to digest first or it

erments on top of previously digested food, leading to indigestion. Fruit at the end of a meal is not a good idea for this
very reason. After eating fruit salad or a piece of fruit, wait
20 minutes before eating anything else.

3 // Fruit does mix with raw greens. Salad with berries or
grilled fruit is a fantastic combination that
is often found on restaurant menus. Green
smoothies also work well if you have access
to them while you're traveling.

Remember, these are guidelines with the
purpose of helping you feel more energetic.
Don't be afraid to experiment with your
own diet. Be sure to notice how you sleep
and how your energy levels are affected as
you try different combinations.

> "ENJOYING AN ESPRESSO
> OR A ROBUST TEA IS
> VERY DIFFERENT FROM
> MAINLINING CAFFEINE
> THROUGHOUT THE DAY
> TO KEEP ON GOING. IN
> LARGE DOSES, CAFFEINE
> INCREASES HEART RATE
> AND RAISES BLOOD
> PRESSURE."

CAFFEINE

Behold the other go-to for energy: caffeine. It is ubiquitous.
Even soft drink giants like Coke and Pepsi have taken note.
Mega-caffeinated drinks are the hottest arrival on the market.
And that is to say nothing of all those fancy coffee outlets that
make a cup of java even more appealing than ever.

Enjoying an espresso or a robust tea is very different from
mainlining caffeine throughout the day to keep on going. In
large doses, caffeine increases heart rate and raises blood pressure. A study in the American Journal of Clinical Nutrition
showed that coffee (not caffeine) consumption raised levels
of homocysteine (an amino acid found in dietary proteins,
usually meat). Research suggests that increased homocysteine

levels may be associated with cardiovascular disease.

Caffeine can increase excretion of stress hormones, which interferes with insulin production. If you're sure you can think better with caffeine, the truth is, it decreases blood flow to the brain by as much as 30%, negatively affecting memory and mental performance.

Caffeine also messes with digestion so I really don't recommend it before or during a flight. A study in *Hepato-Gastroenterology* journal says, "postprandial coffee intake enhances gastric emptying." In other words, coffee helps you go. The study also reports that coffee stimulates gastric emptying of the stomach before food has been digested properly and nutrients absorbed.

Coffee (both decaffeinated and regular) is so strong as a laxative that you may experience constipation if you cut back.

Research shows evidence that caffeine is associated with gastro-esophageal reflux (GERD). In fact, heartburn is the most frequently reported symptom after coffee drinking. Reflux can be very annoying for the traveler so if you have symptoms, cutting back on coffee will be a good start to ameliorating matters.

Caffeine causes depletion of certain minerals, such as calcium, magnesium and potassium, which are all necessary for optimal cellular function. If you have bone density issues and are not consuming sufficient calcium, either cut back on caffeine or increase your calcium intake through legumes, leafy greens, almonds or canned salmon.

Caffeine leads to adrenal fatigue, which has a real impact on your energy. When you drink a cup of coffee, the adrenals are sent a message to release the stress hormones adrenaline and cortisol. (This is the same physiological response as when you are in imminent danger.) Research shows that adrenal response weakens the more coffee you drink in a day, although the occasional cup of coffee has no impact. While you may think you are increasing caffeine tolerance if you're a several-cups-a-day drinker, your adrenals are steadily weakening and not responding as well.

On the flip side, caffeine wakes you up, picks you up, helps concentration and endurance, reduces muscle pain through the release of B-endorphins, stimulates muscles to burn more fat and sugar and has antioxidants that stabilize free radicals so they can't do damage to your cells' DNA.

There's no question that caffeine shouldn't be a prop to help you through your day. If you adjust your diet to include less sugar and dairy, you won't need caffeine as much. Here are some hints for cutting back.

TIPS FOR MANAGING CAFFEINE INTAKE

★ Espresso has less caffeine (more evidence that Italians do it right), and a quick fix might be all you need. A two-ounce double espresso has about 80 milligrams of caffeine compared with 120 milligrams in a 12-ounce brewed cup.

★ Like most things in life, coffee's quality is more important than its quantity. Look for freshly ground, organic beans.

★ Be careful with decaf as usually a chemical process is used to remove the caffeine; look for steam-processed decaffeinated.

★ Watch for hidden caffeine in soft drinks and some medications.

★Withdraw carefully to avoid headaches, constipation and drowsiness. Cut down gradually, preferably over a weekend when it doesn't matter if you hit a wall. Drink plenty of water.

★Avoid using coffee as a receptacle for lots of dairy and sugar.

★For a coffee substitute, try a barley-based drink such as Teeccino.

DAIRY

Can cheese really be an energy kicker? Come on, when did you ever see a cow do anything energetic? Seriously, cheese consumption increases blood sugar. Milk contains a lot of sugar (lactose) and research has shown that drinking one glass of milk can spike insulin levels by 300 percent.

Generally, milk isn't viewed as a high-energy food. Infants are said to be in a milk coma after being breastfed. A cup of warm milk has long been dished up to lull restless folks to sleep. In 1981, researchers discovered morphine in cow and human milk in very mild doses, although the source isn't clear (i.e. were these poppy-consuming cows or medicated humans?). Other opioids such as exorphins are present in milk.

Researchers believe that the opiates have a calming effect on the infant (human or bovine) and nurture the mother-infant bond. According to Dr. Neal Barnard in *Breaking The Food Seduction*, the mildly opiate effect of the milk keeps the baby coming back to feed as it seeks the nutrients it needs.

The protein in cow's milk is called casein, which releases opiates called casomorphins. When cow's milk is made into cheese, the casein is concentrated because of its action on enzymes that would otherwise decrease levels of these opiates. Cow's milk also contains phenylethylamine (PEA) which is an amphetamine-like chemical found in other foods such as sausage and chocolate. Thankfully, cheese isn't about to be classified as a recreational drug.

The message is, if you want to stay awake, skip the cheese sandwich. If you don't want to wave goodbye to cheese altogether (and who would?), use it as a condiment such as shredded parmesan on pasta. Alternatively, enjoy a small portion of good quality cheese after dinner, comme les français. An ounce of Roquefort is worth a pound of "plastic" cheese on a deli sandwich.

ALCOHOL

The days of the three-martini lunch or bottle of wine at a business lunch seem to have been gone for years (how I miss the '80s!), and drinking at breakfast is generally frowned upon, so you're more likely to be indulging in the evening. Since alcohol is a mighty zapper of energy, that's most likely for the best.

That said, while a couple of drinks may make you feel drowsy, that's all it may take to interrupt your sleep pattern, leaving you tired the next day. Overconsumption can lead not just to a lethargy-inspiring hangover, but stinky stale alcohol breath, which colleagues may not appreciate. Furthermore, alcohol stresses the kidneys and adrenal glands, which leads to fatigue.

Abstaining from alcohol can be tough on the road, especially if you're expected to entertain clients. Nothing says you have to go along with peer pressure and there are plenty of people who abstain, even in the alcoholic beverage industry, believe it or not.

In the event that you find yourself boozing mid-week, here are some tips for keeping the after-effects to a minimum.

★ Not only is beer super caloric, it is very high on the glycemic index.

★ Make your first drink a soft one so you don't drink on an empty stomach. Alcohol enters the blood stream really quickly, and sleepiness follows accordingly.

> "NOT ONLY IS BEER SUPER CALORIC, IT IS VERY HIGH ON THE GLYCEMIC INDEX. ...SPIRITS TEND TO BE LIGHTER IN CARBS, BUT THEY ARE HIGH IN ALCOHOL, WHICH WILL STILL DEPLETE ENERGY AS IT ENTERS THE BLOODSTREAM."

★ Wine pairs best with food, so wait until your meal has been served before you have a glass and you won't feel the soporific effects of the alcohol so quickly.

★ Worried about hanging out for the pre-prandial cocktail? Have sparkling water with a slice of lemon and BS with the best of them.

★ Spirits tend to be lighter in carbs, but they are high in alcohol, which will still deplete energy as it enters the bloodstream.

★ Sodas and juices are a major source of hidden sugar, so stick to club soda for a mixer.

★ Spice it up a bit. Club soda is healthier than tonic water but vodka and soda is quite dull. A spicy Bloody Mary or a pepper-flavored vodka with soda and a good squeeze of lime is infinitely more interesting.

★ Always have at least one glass of water per drink; two are better.

★ Whatever you decide, pick your poison, stick to your limits and enjoy.

ADRENAL FATIGUE

Energy lulls can be associated with adrenal fatigue, which affects the thyroid. Daily living is stressful, and stress is tough on the adrenal glands. "The main purpose of your adrenals is to enable your body to deal with stress from every possible source, ranging from injury and disease to work and relationship problems. They largely determine the energy of your body's responses to every change in your internal and external environment." (www.adrenalfatigue.org).

When the adrenals are tired, a variety of symptoms may occur, including low blood sugar, low stamina, low blood pressure, lack of libido, poor sleep patterns and feelings of exhaustion. Make sure your adrenal glands are happy because they are important to a healthy immune system and necessary for proper thyroid function.

How do you keep your adrenal glands happy?

Start by resting and trying to sleep. Business dinners don't always make for early nights, but do your best to make up for it on nights when you're not working. If you've already ditched sugary and processed foods, you're well on your way to strengthening your adrenals. One of their jobs is to help regulate blood sugar levels so ditching the spikes and drops will save them from overworking.

Keep your diet as clean as possible, as you've learned thus far.

Choose quality animal proteins, fresh veggies and fruit, whole grains, legumes and nuts. A clean and simple diet means happy adrenals. Drink plenty of water every day and keep coffee consumption down. The adrenals and kidneys work together, and both love to be flushed with plenty of water.

These *Mile High and Healthy* strategies work. They're based on extensive research and years of personal experience. Some of these tips will leave you feeling energized right away. Others take time before you feel the results. Travel is brutal, but apply all of these steps in combination and you'll be amazed.

CHAPTER 5

JET LAG AND
JET STRESS

When I tell people that I'm traveling transatlantic, the next reaction after "You're so lucky!" is "How do you handle the jet lag?"

Jet lag is the party pooper of international travel. Crossing time zones will cost you more than the price of the globe-spanning ticket. For the business traveler on a tight schedule where performance at a peak level is a necessity, jet lag can be enemy number one. You have to be ready to roll as soon as you land, even if flying from New York to London, or Los Angeles to Miami, on a red-eye. For the leisure traveler, jet lag can ruin the first week of a much-anticipated vacation.

Jet lag, a.k.a. desynchronosis and circadian dysrhythmia, occurs when your circadian rhythms are out of sync. "Circadian rhythms" are up there with "electrolytes" and "immune system" as terms that are bandied around to the point it is assumed we all know what they mean.

I'll let the National Institute of General Medical Sciences do the honors: "Circadian rhythms are physical, mental and behavioral changes that follow a roughly 24-hour cycle, responding primarily to light and darkness in an organism's environment"

> "JET LAG IS THE PARTY POOPER OF INTERNATIONAL TRAVEL. CROSSING TIME ZONES AND SPANNING THE GLOBE WILL COST YOU MORE THAN THE PRICE OF THE TICKET. FOR THE BUSINESS TRAVELER WITH A TIGHT SCHEDULE WHERE PERFORMANCE AT A PEAK LEVEL IS A NECESSITY, JET LAG CAN BE ENEMY NUMBER ONE."

When you jet through multiple time zones and find yourself located five hours ahead in time compared with your point of origin, your circadian rhythms start grumbling: "Wait! Hang on! We need to catch up with you! Why is it dark when it's supposed to be light and light when it's supposed to be dark? We're confused!"

In order to calm your circadian rhythms, let's have a look at the science of how they work.

The SCN (suprachiasmatic nuclei) are the command centers for circadian rhythms. They are located in the anterior hypothalamus at the base of the brain, just above the optic chiasm where visual input from the ambient light/dark cycle is routed to the visual cortex at the back of the brain. Translation: the SCN try to figure out the light/dark conundrum and resynchronize while you experience all kinds of symptoms like poor sleep, brain fog, headaches, grumpiness, bloating, constipation and lack of appetite.

Then there's jet stress, often confused with jet lag, which is the result of the stressful effects of travel: dehydration, travel fatigue, stiffness from lack of movement and potential backaches from cramped seating.

Jet lag recovery time is usually determined by the direction of travel and the number of time zones crossed. According to the Center for Disease Control, with eastward flights, jet lag lasts for the number of days roughly equal to two-thirds the number of time zones crossed. With westward flights the number of days is roughly half the number of time zones. So if you're going from Miami to Paris, which is a change of six time zones, your recovery time would be four days. Your return recovery would be three days.

Those numbers add up to total exhaustion for the business traveler. But there are strategies that can radically alter the effects. Jet lag is real, but it doesn't have to dictate your quality of life. Imagine arriving without immense fatigue, without belly bloat, without brain fog. And imagine all this without recourse to quick fixes in the form of caffeine, sleeping pills and melatonin supplements—none of which is conducive to a traveling lifestyle of any duration.

Lifestyle is the key word. If you are a serial traveler, avoiding jet lag means incorporating changes into your routine so that jet lag-free becomes the norm. Jet lag expert and author of *Farewell Jet Lag; Cures from a Flight Attendant*, Christopher Babayode, sums it up perfectly: "In the present day global economy jet lag is a challenge that requires a lifestyle solution on the part of frequent fliers. No other solution has the scope or longevity to return lasting benefits to the individual or the corporations they serve. Acting on this distinction is the competitive advantage for today's business traveler."

The good news is that these new habits are free and simple. Let's get started.

STAY HYDRATED

Dehydration is a result of flying that can contribute strongly to the body's ability to function efficiently at a cellular level. If you want to avoid brain fog, an upset stomach or lethargy after a flight, being well hydrated will make a huge difference.

While most people know that they should be downing plenty of water during a flight, many don't want to because they dread repeatedly getting up to use the bathroom. Ironically, they might order a soft drink or alcohol instead, which will dehydrate them even more while increasing the volume in the bladder because both caffeine and alcohol are diuretics. Getting up to use the bathroom may be an inconvenience, but intensified jet lag due to dehydration is a deal-breaker. Here's why you want that bottle of water.

Air is drawn into the aircraft cabin from outside. At high altitude, there is no humidity, hence the subsequent drop in cabin humidity to anywhere between 5–20%. In this dry air, you might sense scratchy eyes or an itchy nose, but chances are that your hypothalamus (cool name for the organ that tells you when you're hungry or thirsty) hasn't sent you the thirsty message yet. Also, on terra firma, you lose about 500 milliliters of water through insensible perspiration daily while at rest. That amount is increased in dry air. And because it's insensible, you don't notice.

Fluid loss of just 1% is enough for your body to become dehydrated. While this dryness may lead to a two- to three-pound weight loss per passenger, it's far from a great diet, because of what is happening inside your body.

It is very important to note the color of your urine. Actually, I recommend keeping an eye on it regularly. As you dehydrate, your urine gets darker and darker before you start to behaviorally replace fluid by drinking. The issue is that the hypothalamus takes a while to send the "help, I'm thirsty" signal fast enough. If you drink almost anything other than water at this time, you will most likely exacerbate the situation.

If you don't hydrate, the fluid that your cells need must come from somewhere and that would be from your greatest fluid

MY HIGHLY TECHNICAL METHODOLOGY FOR MONITORING URINE IS AS FOLLOWS:

If your urine is clear or looks like pinot grigio, you're okay.	If it looks like chardonnay, time to ditch the coffee and switch to water.	If it looks like pale ale, time to glug a couple of pints of water.	If it looks like dark ale, put this book down and go and get your kidneys checked right now!

stores—the intracellular fluid. That leaves thirsty cells which means fatigue and poor performance. Dehydration can lead to depressed consciousness, fatigue, muscle weakness, dizziness and cognitive impairment.

That is why the first order of action is always to drink as much water as you can onboard—at least eight ounces for every hour in flight. If you're bothered about having to clamber over a neighbor or needing to go when the fasten seat belt light is on, book an aisle seat to avoid disturbing anyone and making your restroom trips faster.

Another trick is to hydrate like crazy before you fly, while you're still in the terminal and have plenty of access to facilities. So if you're stopping off to have a salad before your flight (see below), glug a few glasses of water with it. Hit the H_2O again when you land.

Unless you're in premium class, you won't see the beverage cart that often so pop to the galley where you'll gladly be given more water (at least on most civilized airlines), or take your own onboard.

// HANDY HINT //

To avoid paying extortionate fees for bottled water from an airport concession, invest in a refillable bottle with a filter. Actually, it's not a big investment because they're very reasonably priced. My favorite is the Bobble Bottle ($11.99 for a 22-ounce bottle), and I don't leave home without it. You can take it through security empty, then fill it from a water fountain because it has a nifty filter built in. These bottles are also ideal if you're heading to a destination that doesn't have potable water.

AVOID ALCOHOL

If you're going on your annual European vacation, and you've used all of your air-miles to upgrade to first class, I get it. Chances are you're going to eat and drink everything in front of you, and watch as many movies as you can while propped up in your lie-flat bed. This is the start of your well-earned holiday, after all.

If work is the main purpose of your trip, however, you want to keep your head as clear as you possibly can. The frequently traveling CEOs and titans of industry that I know do not imbibe as they criss-cross time zones. They know better. Alcohol is extremely dehydrating, as you know if you've ever had too much red wine of an evening and your mouth tastes like sawdust the next morning.

Relaxing with a brew or two before your flight is hard to resist because airport concessions can be appealing places to hang out. Or you might have membership to an airline club that serves complimentary drinks. Nervous flyers often rely on drinks to help them relax. Whatever your reasons, it's very easy to knock a couple back in the club or bar, then have a few more on the flight. If you really must, try to keep it to one and be done. And be sure to soften the harmful side effects of alcohol by drinking plenty of water.

Dehydration aside, your cells are getting their tiny asses whipped by the physical effects of flying; after a drink, they have no chance. Oh, and let's not forget that alcohol totally messes up sleep patterns, too. You're likely to wake up during the night to hit the loo and not be able to get back to sleep.

CUT OUT CAFFEINE

I don't have to tell you that caffeine is a standard pick-me-up, but you should avoid it inflight because it dehydrates wickedly and it can upset the stomach.

Bear in mind that thirst isn't the only symptom of dehydration. Caffeine is a diuretic, which means it increases urination. This is the exact opposite of what you want to happen during a flight or a long car ride.

EAT RIGHT FOR YOUR FLIGHT

Have you ever gotten off a flight feeling and looking like the Michelin Man? I used to think that belly bloat after a long flight was "traveler's tummy," but I've learned it has a scientific name: abdominal barotrauma. As the plane ascends and cabin pressure decreases, intestinal gas expands. Don't you know it as you have to unbuckle your belt, your belly distends and you realize that you are truly full of wind? You may even experience abdominal pain.

Of course, there's an easy way to get rid of gas. You know what it is. However, flatulence fests aren't the most practical of parties to have on a plane. Chances are you're going to resist your body's natural urges, suffer in silence and float off the plane like Violet Beauregarde in *Charlie and the Chocolate Factory.*

Ideally you want to avoid having this unpleasant experience in the first place. This can be done by sticking to a regular healthy diet. (Regular, get it?)

8 TIPS
FOR AVOIDING BELLY BLOAT (ABDOMINAL BAROTRAUMA)

1 // **Ironically, the foods that keep everything up and running can be the ones that cause gas in the first place:** legumes, beans, fresh fruit and vegetables and especially leafy greens. If you are not accustomed to eating a high-fiber diet ("plant based" is the nom du jour), introduce these foods gradually. You may find legumes particularly difficult, which is why Beano was invented, but rather than resort to a supplement, I suggest trying beans one tablespoon at a time until you can digest them more easily. You may find that lentils have a less drastic effect than beans, so they are a good choice for an initial foray into fiber. And please, even I draw the line at Brussels sprouts before a flight.

2 // **Eat a salad before you fly.** If you're not sure about airport offerings, bring your own (stuff leafy greens in a whole-wheat pita to keep it simple). Leafy greens oxygenate the blood, are easy on the digestive system and contain water so they are a good antidote to dehydration as well as barotrauma. A good salad will alkalize your system somewhat before the acidic experience of flying caused by stress, the cabin environment and your physical environment.

3 // **Order a vegan meal if you're dining inflight.** A high-fiber entrée will be easier to digest than the saturated fat and animal protein found in the chicken or beef.

4 // **Pick up chopped fruit or veggies at the airport.** (Better yet, take your own). These whole foods deliver not only fiber, but water and electrolytes, too.

5 // **Avoid the inflight salty nuts and snacks which mess with cellular water content.** Similarly, watch out for salt in drinks like tomato juice, V8 and Bloody Mary mix.

6 // **Be aware that soda and sparkling water can cause discomfort as gas expands in your body.** There's enough of this going on already!

7 // **Take your time while eating.** Your organs are already struggling with inflight conditions and need to be shown a little kindness. Do them a favor by chewing well, resting and digesting.

8 // **Avoid chewing gum midair because you may swallow more air as you masticate.** Please don't chew gum anyway; doing so stresses the jaw.

MANAGE ELECTROLYTE BALANCE

As stated earlier, electrolytes are a buzz-word nowadays. Anyone who works out knows the importance of electrolytes, as evidenced by reliance on Gatorade or coconut water. It's not simply hype. Electrolytes are a major component of health.

Electrolytes are ionized salts (minerals) found in body fluids and the bloodstream in minuscule amounts. They include calcium, magnesium, potassium, sodium, phosphorus, bicarbonate and chloride. When dissolved in water, electrolytes can conduct an electric current. Simply put, electrolytes are the "on/off" switches for the cells. They have a hugely important job to do especially when it comes to the heart, nerves and muscles which rely on electrical activity initiated by electrolytes to function properly.

What does this have to do with jet stress? When you're dehydrated, electrolyte levels in the intracellular and extracellular fluid compartments become unbalanced. Aside from the fact that this can have serious consequences, including cardiac arrest and coma, if your on/off switches aren't functioning properly, you are likely to experience the brain fog and grogginess that accompany jet lag.

> "THE FREQUENT TRAVELING CEO'S AND TITANS OF INDUSTRY THAT I KNOW DO NOT IMBIBE AS THEY CRISSCROSS TIME ZONES. THEY KNOW BETTER."

You might decide to drink lots of water so you can rehydrate and set everything straight. Problem is, we no longer drink water that has picked up minerals from stones as it runs through a swirling, ionizing stream. If you're on a plane, you're probably drinking filtered water which unfortunately, dilutes any electrolytes left in your system. You can't win can you? Well, you can if you cheat a little by taking electrolytes while you fly.

I'm not referring to sports drinks because they are often laced with sugar in some form, and what's with the freaky colors that scream artificial additives? These drinks are designed to give an "energy" boost to someone who has just worked out, hence the added sugar, glucose or fructose.

There are sugar-free electrolyte supplements available such as electroBlast which is recommended by many pilots and cabin crew. I use Emergen-C because the sachets are easy to pack in hand luggage. It has a little sugar, but nothing like Gatorade. I take Emergen-C the morning of an overnight flight, one during flight and one on landing.

Coconut water is a good natural source of electrolytes and worth grabbing if you find some at an airport store. I've even seen it in some hotel minibars.

GATE CHECK YOUR STRESS

You may have had to rush for your flight, or you may have been waiting hours for it. You might be preoccupied with work or family matters. Your preflight condition influences how well you are going to handle your experience above the clouds. If you're agitated, your body automatically hops into fight-or-flight mode. You'll have a harder time sleeping because your cortisol levels are elevated. Your digestive system, usually controlled by the rest-and-digest system, will be overridden by the fight-or-flight system, slowing it down so you lose your appetite. The calmer you remain, the better your body can recover from jet stress.

EXERCISE

Preparing for healthy flying is an ongoing process. At the end of the day, the traveler who is stronger, fitter and healthier will recover more quickly and easily from jet lag and jet stress. Overall health aside, there are two very specific reasons to exercise when crossing time zones.

First, exercise gets the heart pounding and raises the rate of blood circulation in the body. Oxygen is carried via the blood to the brain where it can check in with the SCN (suprachiasmatic nuclei) which ultimately control sleeping patterns.

Secondly, core temperature is another biological rhythm affected by changes in time zones. Circadian rhythms come in two flavors: endogenous (endo = inside) and exogenous (exo = outside). Exogenous rhythms include activity, eating and social contact. Basically, you can decide how and when they occur so you can control them easily and help influence the sleep-wake rhythms.

Core temperature is an endogenous rhythm and adjusts much more slowly to the new time zone. By exercising as part of your jet lag recovery (and hopefully part of your regular routine), you can raise your core temperature to help resynchronize. Research has shown that raising the core temperature in the evening results in increased delta sleep (the deepest slumber we experience). A little pre-bedtime workout followed by a hot bath or shower will help you resynchronize your sleeping pattern.

EAT AT THE RIGHT TIME

Eating is an exogenous rhythm that you can use to manipulate your resynchronization at a new time zone. The SCN cells receive direct input from the retina, which is why they are so responsive to the ambient day/night light rhythm. The input with which these SCN neurons are synchronized is largely affected by, among other things, body temperature (see above) and feeding behavior.

Relative to neuronal and hormonal changes, you have a lot of control over when you eat. Try to adapt to the appropriate meal times at your destination to nudge along the SCN syn-chronization.

GET OUTSIDE

If jet lag is caused by the body not adjusting to light/dark sequences that are out of whack with its internal clock, it makes sense that getting outdoors into bright light might help adjust the body clock to the new time zone.

Research from Flinders University, Australia, tells us that light is the strongest time cue/stimulus for realigning sleep-wake patterns, "This re-times the body clock to enable daytime alertness and good sleep at night time. In the case of flying westward, as from Australia to Europe, to get over the jet lag in Europe your body clock needs to be delayed.... However, in Europe these same hours with respect to your body clock will be late afternoon. Therefore, getting light stimulation from the early afternoon for as long as sunlight is available will help you get over jet lag more quickly."

Some experts specify times to be outside while you're adjusting. Practicality says the business traveler is going to fit in whatever he or she can per work schedules. Leisure travelers have more opportunity when out and about sight-seeing or sitting on a beach. Make the most of what is available to you.

If you're traveling east you can start to adapt to your new time zone by waking up an hour earlier for a few days before you fly and getting exposure to sunlight. You don't want to get up too much earlier or you'll be messed up on current times and the sun may not have risen.

Going east to west is easier because our natural circadian rhythms are just over 24 hours. The longer day you experience by going back in time, as it were, makes for an easier adjustment as long as you can stay awake until a regular bedtime for that zone. I find if I can make it to 9 p.m. without napping, I'll get a full night's sleep and not wake up ridiculously early. Of course, time spent outside will help, too. The earlier the new light/dark cycle is experienced, the sooner the resynchronization of circadian rhythms will occur.

GET GROUNDED

This is where you might think I'm slightly nuts. A couple of years ago I was struggling with jet lag after a flight from Orlando to Milan via Frankfurt. I'd ordered a vegan meal, I was eating salads left, right and center, and if I'd drunk any more water, I would have burst. I made a quick call to my pal, Christopher Babayode, author of *Farewell Jet Lag: Cures from a Flight Attendant*, who told me to go earthing or grounding, as the practice is often known.

I know what you're thinking. What the heck is earthing or grounding?

Chris wanted me to go and stand barefooted on grass, sand or cement for at least twenty minutes so I could connect with the Earth. After donning a muumuu and a tied-dyed scarf (kidding!), I found a patch of grass outside the Castello Sforzesco, checked for dog poop and kicked off my shoes.

Seems weird, right? Well, I slept like a log that night, and every time I fly transatlantic now, I add grounding to my arsenal of jet lag-combatting tools. I appreciate that my experience is anecdotal rather than scientifically proven, so I was anxious to learn more. I came across Clint Ober, Stephen T. Sinatra and Martin Zucker's book *Earthing: The Most Important Health Discovery Ever?* and the Earthing Institute. Both provide anecdotes with plenty of hallelujah moments about the health benefits of earthing and the results of a few scientific studies. Earthing is still not exactly mainstream, so just what is it about?

Humans are electrical beings. Every cell in the body has electrical properties. The body regularly produces positive charges, which can be harmful if they oxidize or if there are too many of them. The Earth's surface is just the opposite; it has a negative charge and an unlimited supply of free electrons. When you stand barefoot on the Earth, you become a conductor, or an antenna, that sucks up free electrons to balance the positive charges in your body.

> "WHEN YOU STAND BAREFOOT ON THE EARTH, YOU BECOME A CONDUCTOR, OR AN ANTENNA, THAT SUCKS UP FREE ELECTRONS TO BALANCE THE POSITIVE CHARGES IN YOUR BODY."

The theory is that we ended up in this mess in the first place because we've lost our connection with the Earth. We wear shoes, our buildings no longer have earth flooring, some of us live in multistory housing and, not to be overlooked, we fly in tin cans over 30,000 feet above the Earth. The California Institute of Human Sciences conducted an experiment which demonstrated that the human body checks for its reference to the Earth every 90 seconds.

"At any point on the surface of the planet, the Earth's energy potential fluctuates according to the position of the sun and the moon, creating cycles such as the circadian cycle," the authors of *Earthing* explain. "This understanding helps to explain how passengers, after long flights across many time zones, can reset their internal clocks to 'local time,' so to speak, and quickly reduce the effect of jet lag by going barefoot or grounding themselves after arriving at their destination." They further hypothesize that the rhythm of melatonin—the sleep-promoting factor—is normalized while sleeping grounded.

A 2007 study published in the *Journal of Alternative and Complementary Medicine* states: "The most reasonable hypothesis to explain the beneficial effects of earthing is that a direct earth connection enables both diurnal electrical rhythms and free electrons to flow from the earth to the body. It is proposed that the earth's diurnal electrical rhythms set the biological clocks for hormones that regulate sleep and activity."

There is no doubt that more research is needed about earthing. In the meantime, why don't you try it and form your own opinion? It's free and it's simple, after all. That said, if you're stuck in a snow storm or can't find a suitable patch of ground on which to go barefoot, you can purchase grounding sheets and mats online. Many people travel with their earthing sheet to ensure speedy jet lag recovery.

CHAPTER 6

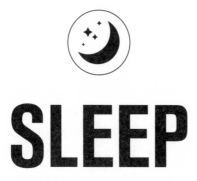

SLEEP

A global well-being survey conducted by Westin Hotels & Resorts in 2014 revealed: "After a stressful workday, 40% of global business travelers said they would prefer sleep over sex." No one who travels regularly would be surprised.

The fact is, there are not many people who get enough sleep in any walk of life, but sleep deprivation for road warriors is endemic, part and parcel of a culture of high achievement and a "get the job done at all costs" mentality. When you factor in the various conditions of constant travel—all of which are destructive to healthy sleep—you have a recipe for disaster.

No one is more detached from the natural 24-hour cycles of light and dark than road warriors who cross time zones and have to acclimate to different places all over the planet. Long days and long nights are difficult enough, but throw jet lag into the equation and it's even worse.

> "LONG DAYS AND LONG NIGHTS ARE DIFFICULT ENOUGH, BUT THROW JET LAG INTO THE EQUATION AND IT'S EVEN WORSE. … FACTORS OF INTEREST TO TRAVELERS ARE DECREASED PERFORMANCE AND ALERTNESS, LACK OF CONCENTRATION, COMPROMISED COMMUNICATION AND DECISION-MAKING, ANXIETY, DEPRESSION AND MOOD FLUCTUATION."

The consequences of sleep deprivation are profound. Memory function, weight maintenance and damage to your immune system are only a few of the negative impacts—chronic lack of sleep also leaves you vulnerable to serious conditions, such as cardiovascular disease, diabetes and certain types of cancer. Other factors of interest to travelers are decreased performance and alertness, lack of concentration, compromised communication and decision-making, anxiety, depression and mood fluctuation.

When you're tired, it's nearly impossible to judge your own level of impairment. That puts you at risk for all kinds of accidents, including driving while sleep deprived, veering off the road in otherwise good conditions or falling asleep at the wheel.

Being awake is part of being fit for duty. You can't catch up from sleep deprivation on the weekends; it is regulated daily. Here's how to start sleeping better right now.

HOW TO SLEEP BETTER WITHOUT POTIONS OR PILLS

Eat Light. Late, heavy dinners can be par for the course for business travelers. You're having a dinner meeting; arriving late at your destination after a flight with no meal service, you're starving, your willpower is shot and, being exhausted, it's easy to convince yourself a calorie-fest of rich food will make you feel better. If you don't have a dinner meeting, you're still going to face temptation. Again, tired and hungry, you pick up the room service menu and the compulsion to feast is sometimes overwhelming, especially since you may have been getting by on airline snacks for hours

But long heavy meals are sleep killers. They're harder to digest, usually taking up to 40 hours to journey through the digestive tract. (Think that's bad? A typical Christmas dinner takes about 72 hours.)

On a regular night, your liver helps with digesting and detoxing typically between the hours of 10 p.m. and 2 a.m. The more help you can offer the liver in this process, the better. Keep your meal light so it digests more easily. Squeeze as many veggies as possible onto your plate with a small serving of animal protein or pasta and a simple sauce. Avoid large servings of meat, dairy, rich sauces and overly spicy dishes, all factors that will leave you restless and bloated as your stomach gurgles away.

Try to consume the heaviest part of your meal before 8 p.m. That way, you have time to digest, keep alcohol to a minimum and avoid dessert. If you're in a country where dinner is typically served late in the evening (in Spain, supper starts at 10 o'clock at night), eat as light as you can. Keep a ginger tea packet in your bag for post-prandial help with digestion.

If you're on an overnight flight, dinner is often served later than your time zone of origin and in the middle of the night at your destination. Many top-performing executives eat before they fly, taking advantage of their airlines' premium service clubs and decline inflight meals altogether so they can work or sleep on the plane. If that's not happening for you, take my previous advice and order a vegetarian meal.

Recent research reported in *Acta Pharmaceutica Sinica B* (the journal of the Chinese Pharmaceutical Association and Institute of Materia Medica, Chinese Academy of Medical Sciences) has shown evidence that the liver has its own hepatic circadian clock, operating independently of the SCN (suprachiasmatic nucleus). That means it's got its own deal going on, its own little circadian rhythm, largely regulated by the patterns of food intake (as opposed to the SCN which is largely influenced by light). Disruption in meal times throws off the hepatic circadian clock and leads to dysfunction of regular liver activity, including digestion. Regulating the timing of meals to match your destination means maintenance of the normal hepatic circadian clock, which communicates to the SCN that all is right in the world. When that's the case, normal sleep patterns will ensue.

Avoid sugary foods. Eating sugary foods will spike blood glucose levels and have you bouncing off the walls before bed. This will put you on a hamster's wheel with no way off, because the lack of sleep itself then affects insulin production.

A 1999 report in *The Lancet* explained that sleep deprivation affected the body's ability to control both blood sugar and cortisol levels leading to a harmful impact on carbohydrate metabolism and endocrine function. This means that lack of sleep can contribute to weight gain and, as the study explained, "Sleep debt may increase the severity of age-related chronic disorders."

Avoid alcohol. While alcohol may send you to sleep, it also interrupts sleep patterns, particularly in the latter part of the night when you might wake up and not be able to fall back into a slumber until it's time to start your day.

A 2015 study in *Alcoholism: Clinical and Experimental Research* confirmed that having a drink before bed did increase slow-wave sleep and delta wave (deepest slumber) activity. This is when you nod off into a deep sleep after a drink or three. However, the research also showed a simultaneous increase in alpha waves (least sleepy, most active).

> "WHILE ALCOHOL MAY SEND YOU TO SLEEP, IT ALSO INTERRUPTS SLEEP PATTERNS.... THE STUDY CONFIRMED THAT ALCOHOL CAUSES THIS DISRUPTION AND AFFECTS CONSEQUENT DAYTIME FUNCTIONING. THE EFFECTS OF ALCOHOL ON SLEEP DISRUPTION CAN BE CUMULATIVE IF NIGHT-TIME CONSUMPTION IS A REGULAR HABIT."

Delta and alpha waves do not usually hang out together during normal sleep. When they do, disruptive stimuli present themselves and the pattern is interrupted. The study confirmed that alcohol causes this disruption and affects consequent daytime functioning. The effects of alcohol on sleep disruption can be cumulative if night time consumption is a regular habit.

Cut out caffeine. This might seem a bit obvious, but it's good to know how little caffeine you actually need to stay awake, how much more you probably consume throughout the day and the effect it has on your sleeping patterns. An eight-ounce cup of coffee contains around 100 milligrams of caffeine. If you have that at 8 a.m., you will still have 25 milligrams left in your body 12 hours later. That's right, one regular cup of coffee at eight in the morning means you'll still have 12.5 milligrams of caffeine in your system at bed time. To put this in perspective, to keep awake, you only need about 20 milligrams of caffeine every two hours. The average person drinks three 12-ounce cups of coffee on weekdays.

"THAT'S RIGHT, ONE REGULAR CUP OF COFFEE AT EIGHT IN THE MORNING MEANS YOU'LL STILL HAVE 12.5 MILLIGRAMS OF CAFFEINE IN YOUR SYSTEM AT BEDTIME. TO PUT THIS IN PERSPECTIVE, TO KEEP AWAKE, YOU ONLY NEED ABOUT 20 MILLIGRAMS OF CAFFEINE EVERY TWO HOURS."

If you think caffeine doesn't affect you, you're probably wrong. Better to skip the postprandial coffee.

Time your water intake. Staying hydrated is vital, but it's very important to time your water consumption so you avoid nocturia, or excessive urinating at night.

My best recommendation is that you drink as much water as you can first thing in the morning when it is easier to take in because you're naturally dehydrated at that time.

Let's say you want to have about two liters or 64 ounces of water per day. Make sure you have an eight-ounce glass by your bed so you drink it as soon as you wake up, have another glass before you have your coffee or tea, and one or more while you get ready for work. I strongly recommend having half your daily total before you leave the house. The other advantage here is that while you're doing this as part of your morning routine, you're close to a bathroom so it won't be a big deal if you have to use the loo more frequently.

Aim to have most of your water by 4 p.m. and just one glass or so over the course of dinner. Absolutely no water for an hour before you go to bed.

Exercise. As invigorated as one feels after working out, research shows that exercise is an attractive antidote for insomnia. Dr. Shawn Youngstedt in a 2005 article in *Clinics in Sports Medicine* writes, "Hypotheses that sleep serves an energy conservation function, a body tissue restitution function, or a temperature down-regulation function all have predicted a uniquely potent effect of exercise on sleep because no other stimulus elicits greater depletion of energy stores, tissue breakdown, or elevation of body temperature, respectively."

Raise your body temperature. A 1988 study at the University of California showed that raising body temperature in the early or late evening is conducive to increasing deep delta sleep and reducing REM (lighter sleep when most dreams occur). An increase in body temperature in the early evening increased delta waves in particular over later sleep cycles. So, a hot shower or soak in the tub prior to turning in for the night is a good way to ensure a solid slumber.

Take a catnap. Okay, not during meetings, but otherwise a quick nap (15 to 20 minutes) can improve alertness and performance for as long as two to three hours. While you might be reluctant to spend time on a nap, your increased productivity will more than compensate.

Have a ritual. A familiar ritual that you can take with you from place to place will help you adapt to sleeping in strange places because it teaches the brain to recognize a routine that heralds a regular sleep time.

The key is to find what works for you and stick to it. For my part, I have a small travel candle I take everywhere I go so that I have the familiar scent in the room. A night time bath, relaxing music, or reading something nonwork related can help, as can meditation if it is your thing. Otherwise, focus the mind by counting sheep, imagining what you'll do with your lottery winnings or kick back and plan your perfect day.

Get rid of lights. The 2011 Sleep in America Poll revealed that 95 of Americans use electronic devices a few nights a week in the hour before bed. Light-emitting screens suppress melatonin, the sleep-inducing hormone, so you're less likely to fall asleep if you're checking emails, texting or watching TV before bed.

The blue light emitted by electronics and energy-efficient lightbulbs suppresses melatonin more than any other type of light. Researchers at Harvard compared the effects of 6.5 hours of exposure to both blue and green light of comparable brightness. They discovered that the blue light suppressed melatonin for about twice as long as green light and shifted circadian rhythms by twice as much (three hours v. 1.5 hours).

You can buy glasses with special lenses that block out only blue light if you're really having trouble sleeping. Alternatively, avoid looking at any electronic screens, including your laptop and the TV, for a couple of hours before going to bed.

Find the right temperature for you. Standard advice is to sleep in a cool room, but respect your individuality. I personally wrap up like I'm in the Arctic Circle at night, whereas other people like a colder room. Find the ambient temperature that suits you to help ensure an uninterrupted night.

Allow 8 to 9 hours for sleep. Guaranteeing a set number of hours for sleep is a luxury that eludes many frequent travelers. Chances are you won't be able to do this every night, but when you can, take advantage. The sooner you catch up on sleep, the better. Being sleep deprived during the week and making up for it on the weekends doesn't work.

Avoid stress before bed. Have you ever checked email "one last time" before bed only to find a disturbing message waiting? Similarly watching the news or a violent TV show can thwart your attempts to sleep or even give you nightmares. Set a time to switch off from media, and stick to it. Messages can wait until the morning.

"THE 2011 SLEEP IN AMERICA POLL REVEALED THAT 95% OF AMERICANS USE ELECTRONICS A FEW NIGHTS A WEEK IN THE HOUR BEFORE BED. LIGHT EMITTING SCREENS SUPPRESS MELATONIN. MELATONIN IS THE SLEEP INDUCING HORMONE, SO YOU'RE LESS LIKELY TO FALL ASLEEP IF YOU'RE CHECKING EMAILS, TEXTING OR WATCHING TV BEFORE BED."

TIPS FOR SLEEPING IN A HOTEL

Cover as many lights as you can. This includes the alarm clock and TV. Use an eye mask as recommended below if needed.

Use earplugs. They block out the noise of the refrigerator and any hallway activity.

Consider a white noise app. Good ones such as Sleep Miracle or Rain, Rain, will mask background noise and lull you to sleep.

Keep the bed clear of clutter. This is important. Your work stuff should be on the desk.

Turn digital devices down or off.

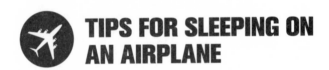

TIPS FOR SLEEPING ON AN AIRPLANE

Go to www.seatguru.com. If you're in first class and have a lie-flat bed—or these days, there are even private cabins—then your chances of sleeping are pretty good. However, if you're with the masses crammed into seats with a 30-inch pitch, well, we've all been there and we know the odds aren't good when it comes to catching Zzzs. The seatguru website can make these odds better.

It's a great website every frequent traveler should investigate. Enter your flight number, and you'll find a seat map for your plane, indicating which are the seats to be avoided. For example, instead of upgrading on a red-eye, I book row 16 or 17 in coach on an American Airlines.

Wear an eye mask. The lights in a plane will keep you awake all night by interrupting melatonin production. Even if the lights are dimmed, you'll still perceive that they're on, and you won't enjoy quality slumber. An eye mask with full coverage will completely block out light and allow you to produce melatonin as you usually would.

I swear by the Lewis N. Clark Comfort Eye Mask. Out of all my *Mile High and Healthy* essential items, this is the one that I take everywhere (I have five just in case I misplace one!). You can buy a two-pack from Amazon.com for about $12.

Stay warm. Airplanes can be cold, especially on overnight flights. Make sure you have warm clothes so you're not kept awake shivering. There aren't always enough blankets on board for each passenger, so you might want to bring a shawl or jacket to cover you.

> "MAKE SURE YOU HAVE WARM CLOTHES SO YOU'RE NOT KEPT AWAKE SHIVERING. THERE AREN'T ALWAYS ENOUGH BLANKETS ON BOARD FOR EACH PASSENGER, SO YOU MIGHT WANT TO BRING A SHAWL OR JACKET TO COVER YOU."

Noise cancelling headphones. These are a wonderful investment. They really do work for blocking out the background din.

WHAT ABOUT MELATONIN?

Melatonin is known as the Dracula hormone because it is only at night that it signals your body that it's dark outside. The role of melatonin on sleep per se is less clear. It is believed that it's the circadian system that opens the sleep gate and switches on melatonin production.

I'm often asked if travelers should take melatonin supplements to help them sleep. The short answer is no. A supplement can induce sleepiness if it is light out, but I prefer to don my fabulous eye mask, blocking out the light so my pineal gland can get to work manufacturing melatonin.

Understand that melatonin supplements are made either from synthetic chemicals or from animal ingredients including cow's urine. There is no ideal substitute for the body's own (endogenous) melatonin, and both "natural" and synthetic supplements have side effects such as dizziness and headaches.

A 2004 study at the University of Alberta concluded that supplemental melatonin was not effective for the treatment of most primary and secondary sleep disorders. It found no evidence of effectiveness for jet lag and shift worker disorders. Another study in the *Sleep Medicine Reviews* the following year stated, "No long-term safety data exist, and the optimum dose and formulation for any application (of melatonin) remains to be clarified."

You can also look to certain food sources for melatonin. A study from Khon Kaen University, Thailand, found that consuming certain tropical fruits raises blood levels of melatonin naturally. Pineapple increased 6-sulfatyoxymelatonin (aMT6s) levels by 266%, banana by 180% and oranges by 47%. Another study found that drinking tart cherry juice for seven days increased sleep by an average of 34 minutes a night and increased sleep efficiency by 5–6%.

Other foods that raise aMT6s levels are oats, sweet corn, rice, ginger, tomatoes, mangosteen and barley. Far more appealing than cow's urine!

CHAPTER 7

HOW TO AVOID GETTING SICK WHILE **TRAVELING**

For me, traveling means trying new cuisines. I'm a hardcore foodie, and that means sampling everything, including street food. It all started in Cairo when I was 19. Living on a student budget, I'd purchase shawarma from a street vendor's cart every night, a practice I continued in the Sudan the next year. My ventures into parts unknown resulted in two bouts of amoebic dysentery, ghiardiasis and three rounds of malaria. (But I can't blame the malaria on the food). Did I learn from this? No. Do I still eat street food? You bet. Whether it's roti in Trinidad, jerk in Jamaica, empanadas in Puerto Rico or tacos in LA, I'm there.

The difference is that I don't get sick any more. I like to think that it's because I have a steel constitution built on the bravura of my youth. I've developed that can't-touch-me attitude that seems common to many frequent travelers. That we have built up some kind of natural resistance to all things disease-inducing.

Actually, what I've done is worked on strengthening my immune system. Everybody has heard about the immune system, but here is another term much used and little understood. In his renowned book, *The China Study*, Dr. T. Colin Campbell writes, "I often hear people speaking about this system as if it were an identifiable organ like a lung. Nothing could be further from the truth. It is a system, not an organ."

A system means many moving and interrelated parts. Consequently, there are a number of components to keeping your immune system healthy. My grandmother called her immune system her "moon system" and was not only aware of it (unusual for someone of her generation) but took steps to protect it. She lived to be 95.

The immune system is a collection of cells, tissues and organs (white blood cells, thymus, bone marrow and

"...THERE ARE A NUMBER OF COMPONENTS TO KEEPING YOUR IMMUNE SYSTEM HEALTHY. MY GRANDMOTHER CALLED HER IMMUNE SYSTEM HER 'MOON SYSTEM,' AND WAS NOT ONLY AWARE OF IT (UNUSUAL FOR SOMEONE OF HER GENERATION) BUT TOOK STEPS TO PROTECT IT. SHE LIVED TO BE 95."

lymph nodes) that work together to provide resistance to infection and toxins. The human body is designed to self-regulate and is constantly seeking balance among all of its systems, a process called homeostasis. If something runs amok at a cellular level, reactions are in place to assist the body in fully restoring and maintaining homeostasis.

This balance is thrown off kilter by infections, stress, poor diet and lack of exercise, all of which provide the free radicals (which are already present and circulating) with the opportunity to interfere with the immune system. Free radicals are volatile molecules that damage cells, which can cause cancer and other diseases.

Travelers are regularly faced with circumstances that may compromise their immune systems: stress, bad food, germs and acidic flying conditions. You get tired, you're exposed to the general public, you sleep in beds that other people have slept in, you have no idea where your food is coming from or how it's being prepared, you don't always have the time to exercise and your circadian rhythms are disrupted.

The good news is that you have substantial control over repairing and sustaining your immune system. Prevention is always better than cure, so follow the steps below to ensure a seamless transition from hotel to home.

Avoid acidic foods that upset the body's pH balance. Acidity leads to inflammation, which is the fundamental cause of most chronic conditions. Acidic foods include meat, dairy, sugar, juices and alcohol. Instead, opt for fruits, vegetables, whole grains and legumes.

Work on getting a good night's sleep as this is when your body repairs itself. Uninterrupted sleep is vital for the liver to carry out its detoxifying functions, thus the fewer toxins, the less likelihood of inflammation. Quality sleep is elusive for many travelers—head back to chapter 6 for advice on how to enjoy more restful slumber.

Keep your blood pressure in check. This is accomplished with a healthy diet and plenty of exercise.

Wash your hands frequently. This will help avoid infection.

Maintain a healthy weight. Toxins hang out in fat cells, so the fewer the better.

Practice preventive medicine. Make time in your schedule to have an annual check-up.

Exercise. Road warriors need to be strong, and that's not going to happen if you don't take the time to exercise. A healthy immune system is part of overall good health which exercise helps achieve through good blood circulation, nourishing the cells and allowing the immune system cells to travel throughout the body doing their magic.

Minimize stress. Frequent travel presents a multitude of opportunities for stress. You can't eliminate the stress, but you can change how you handle and minimize it. Chapter 8 will offer tips to help achieve this.

Don't smoke.

Diet. A healthy diet deserves a separate mention because, like exercise, it is a huge factor for overall health and a strong immune system. According to the website harvard health publications (www.hsph. harvard.edu/prc/publications/): "Like any fighting force, the immune system army marches on its stomach. Immune system warriors need good, regular nourishment." This means a diet that is rich in fruit and vegetables supplemented with good quality protein and high-fiber carbs.

Why the emphasis on fruit and vegetables? Because they are rich in antioxidants and phytochemicals. Certain animal-derived foods have antioxidants, too, but since "phyto" means "plant" you won't find phytochemicals in meat, fish or eggs.

Antioxidants are vitamins and minerals, but just to confuse matters, they can also be phytochemicals. Antioxidants, as the name suggests, attack anything that is "oxidizing" a cell. That would be free radicals, those volatile cell-damaging, disease-causing molecules mentioned earlier. Antioxidants can repair cell damage from acidic substances, such as the foods mentioned above, or from cigarette smoking, environmental toxins, fried foods and more.

> "YOU'LL FIND ANTIOXIDANTS IN FRUIT, VEGETABLES AND LEGUMES.... THAT'S WHY WE'RE TOLD TO EAT A RAINBOW OF COLORS, IN ORDER TO BENEFIT FROM THE MULTITUDE OF ANTIOXIDANTS AVAILABLE IN PLANT FOODS."

You'll find antioxidants in fruit, vegetables and legumes where they are represented as pigments. That's why we're told to eat a rainbow of colors, in order to benefit from the multitude of antioxidants available in plant foods.

Phytochemicals also work to promote good health. Plants make phytochemicals to protect themselves against viruses and bacteria, so when you eat those plants you, too, get the benefits of their protective factors. Beyond general health, research has shown that phyto-chemicals help protect against cancer, heart disease, macular degeneration and other chronic diseases.

Phytochemicals include polyphenols, carotenoids and phytosterols. Of these, polyphenols are divided into biofla-vonoids, tannins and lignans. Tannins keep the digestive system healthy. Lig-nans have hormone-like properties and may help to reduce the risk of cardiovascular disease.

Carotenoids provide Vitamin A and contribute to healthy vision, bolster the immune system and reduce the risk of cardiovascular disease and some cancers. Phytosterols help to reduce symptoms of an enlarged prostrate and are effective for keeping cholesterol levels in check.

WHERE TO FIND ANTIOXIDANTS AND PHYTOCHEMICALS

★ Choose whole foods and vegetables, with the skin on, whenever possible. Phytochemicals and plant fibers are lost in food processing.

★ Bioflavonoids are the pigments in red, blue, pur-ple and black fruits, vegetables and legumes.

★ Tannins are found in tea and are your excuse for enjoying a glass of red wine.

★ Lignans are the cell walls of plants and are stringy in structure, the bits of celery that get stuck in your teeth. You'll find lignans in cereals, peanuts, cashews, peaches, broccoli, winter squash and many seeds, including flax, sesame and sunflower.

★ Carotenoids, of which there are over 600 types, are red, yellow and orange pigments. You'll find them in carrots, tomatoes, sweet potatoes, dark leafy greens, romaine lettuce, cantaloupe, red peppers, dried apricots and so much more.

★ Heard of cholesterol? Of course you have. Phytosterols are the plant equivalent that actually helps reduce "bad" LDL cholesterol. You'll find phytosterols in wheat germ oil, corn oil, rice bran oil and canola, as well as sesame and sunflower seeds, pistachios, pine nuts and almonds. They are also in whole grains such as wheat germ, bran, whole-wheat flour, rye flour, buckwheat flour, soy flour and soybeans. That's a lot of sources, so no excuses for skipping phytosterols.

★ I use the acronym ACES to remember that Vitamins A, C, and E are antioxidants, as well as the trace mineral Selenium, all of which fight cell damage.

★ Vitamin A can be found in carrots and spinach, broccoli, cantaloupe, tomato juice, apricots, sweet potato, pumpkin and collard greens. Animal sources include milk, cheese, egg yolk and liver. Carotenoids are released and absorbed more easily from cooked vegetables than raw.

★ Vitamin C occurs in broccoli, strawberries, kiwi fruit, oranges, tomatoes, watermelon, cabbage, sweet potatoes, sweet peppers and chili peppers.

★ You'll find Vitamin E in nuts, seeds, spinach, vegetable oils, peanut butter, tomatoes, sunflower seeds, red pasta sauce, sardines, dark leafy greens and avocadoes.

★ Good sources of selenium are fish and seafood, legumes, whole grains, lean meats, dairy products and Brazil nuts.

SUPERFOODS

Foods with claims to having extraordinary health properties are called superfoods. In most cases, they are simply fruit and vegetables with high antioxidant content. There is no official definition for superfoods and health claims are not permitted on their packaging in most countries. Where research has been conducted on superfoods, it has usually been done with highly concentrated purified extracts, which is not how they would be normally consumed.

The lack of official acceptance shouldn't stop you from eating a diet rich in antioxidants and phytochemicals, especially in the case of easily available superfoods such as kale, garlic, blue berries, broccoli and green tea.

Every now and again, a new superfood rises to stardom. We've seen it happen with kale, quinoa, pomegranates and açai berries. Understand that no single food can cause miracles. Eat a variety of fresh produce and keep processed foods to a minimum.

6 LESS
MAINSTREAM SUPERFOODS

CHOCOLATE

Yes, chocolate, the food of the Mayan gods. Chocolate contains magnesium, iron, manganese and chromium. It is also mildly (or in my case, massively) addictive because of its theobromine and anandramide content.

Before you jump up and down and add three candy bars a day to your regimen, understand that in most cases, cocoa is combined with saturated fat and sugar to make chocolate, negating many of its health benefits.

Raw chocolate with the fewest ingredients, a high cacao content and devoid of soy lecithin fillers, is your best bet. Vita Chocolate is my recommendation as it has just three basic ingredients and can easily be ordered online at vitaorganicfoods.com. Keep your chocolate serving to the size of a credit card.

GOJI BERRIES

Goji Berries have been used in traditional Chinese medicine for over 5,000 years. They contain 18 different amino acids, 21 trace minerals, iron, vitamins B and E and more. The argument against gojis is that they are expensive, and you might find the same nutrients by eating a variety of cheaper plant foods.

I like to include goji berries as a snack, mixed with raw almonds and raw cacao nibs. As for the price, I figure it balances out with what I save on airport food.

SPIRULINA

Spirulina is a form of cyanobacterium, credited with the highest source of complete protein in the world. Advocates for spirulina purport that it can stabilize blood sugar and help diabetes, but the allopathic community currently rejects those claims. Traditionally, spirulina was consumed by the Aztecs and continues to be harvested in Chad.

Spirulina usually comes in powder form and can be added to smoothies, or you can take it as a supplement. I once put too much in a smoothie and had green teeth for the rest of the day, so be careful.

SEA VEGETABLES

Sea vegetables, such as kelp, dulse, nori, hikki and chlorella, are becoming increasingly popular as sources of plant protein and micronutrients. In fact, sea vegetables are consumed by a number of indigenous populations, and seaweed figures prominently in Japanese cuisine as a principle ingredient of sushi.

Sea vegetables are said to have thyroid boosting and detoxifying properties in addition to a high volume of micronutrients. Add seaweed to your diet as a way of increasing the variety of plant foods you consume. Aside from sushi, you can sprinkle kelp and dulse flakes on salads. Be careful with the bright green seaweed salad that is served at some Japanese restaurants as it often contains artificial coloring and additives. Look for wakame and kombu instead.

HEMP SEEDS

I give hemp seeds thumbs up because they are an easy snack to take on the road. You can purchase individual packets for sprinkling on salad, yogurt and adding to healthy cereals. Check out Hemp Hearts by manitobaharvest.com if you can't find hemp seeds at your supermarket.

Nutritionally, hemp seeds are high in omega-3 fatty acids, iron, vitamin E and amino acids.

CHIA SEEDS

Another high-priced super food! The good news is that you only need a small amount of chia to pack a nutritional punch. The seeds are high in omega-3 fatty acids, B vitamins, calcium, iron, magnesium, manganese, phosphorus and zinc.

Chia seeds can be found in individual serving packets. They are usually added to smoothies or yogurt, a very handy way to consume them if you're on the road. The seeds expand when added to liquid and give a gelatinous consistency, which is a bit odd—but no worse than the semolina pudding I used to get at school lunches.

AIRBORNE ILLNESSES

Travelers often complain about picking up colds or the flu after flying. I've certainly blamed the odd cold on fellow passengers. Confined spaces, reused blankets and pillows plus proximity to other people over the course of several hours mean exposure from breathing, coughing and sneezing as germs are released into the air.

A 2004 study in the *Journal of Environmental Health Research* revealed that 20% of passengers reported colds five to seven days after a two-and-a-half-hour flight.

According to Mariana Calleja, M.D., founder of travelthy. com, "Touch is the most common way to get infected during air travel. For example, everyone without exception has some kind of contact with other people's germs whenever they go to the toilet and grab the door handle, or when they touch seat heads as they walk through the aisle during flight, or when they are talking to a hotel's front desk staff, exchanging documents and waiting with arms on the counter during the check-in process." Dr. Calleja says the simplest way to avoid infection is to wash one's hands as often as possible.

By the way, it's wise to monitor yourself for a few days after a trip because symptoms may not appear immediately. Continue to hydrate and look for signs, such as digestive trouble, unexplained fevers or headaches and skin reactions.

Proximity to others is the primary factor that causes germs to spread. There is a misconception at large that the recirculating air in the cabin is to blame. A 2002 study by the Aerospace Medical Association concluded that there was "no evidence that organisms pass from one person to another through the aircraft ventilation system." Note that in newer aircraft 50% of the air in the cabin is recirculated and passes through filters that remove bacteria, fungi and most viruses. The other 50% of the air comes from outside. These findings were corroborated by further studies in 2010.

So why do people get sick so often after concluding a hectic travel schedule? You got it—travel can imperil the immune system. As we've seen, you're dealing with dry cabin air, potential fatigue and very close and continuous contact with a bunch of other human beings. Your ability to resist infection, thanks to the strength of your immune system, will strongly influence whether or not you catch an infection on a plane.

A 1997 study in the *European Respiratory Journal* suggests that low humidity impairs your ability to resist germs because the mechanism that protects against colds slows down or stops when there is low humidity. This would be your Mucociliary Clearance System, which traps viruses and bacteria before moving them from the nose and throat to destruction in the stomach. When dry, the mucus becomes too thick to be moved by the cilia (little hairs) that normally push it along. The infectious bodies hang around and you get sick. This is another most excellent reason to stay hydrated.

HANDY PRODUCTS TO HELP WARD OFF AIRBORNE INFECTIONS:

GERM WARRIOR. This homeopathic nasal inhaler designed to fight airborne germs and help boost immune defenses.

HALO ORAL ANTISEPTIC. Not your ordinary mouthwash, you spray Halo Oral into your mouth before boarding to decrease airborne pathogens to which you might be exposed.

SAVVY TRAVELER KLEAN OFFZ. These surface wipes are individually wrapped, making them perfect for travel. Use the anti- bacterial wipe to clean the spots where many germs lurk onboard—tray table, armrest and remote control— and to do a once-over of surfaces in your hotel room.

KLEAN UPZ. Also by Savvy Traveler, these antibacterial wipes, are for hand and body use.

EAR BAROTRAUMA

The abdomen isn't the only body cavity that fills with gas when cabin pressure decreases during take-off and increases during landing (see Chapter 5); the middle ear and sinuses are affected too.

The ear is especially susceptible when the eustachian tubes (ear passages) are blocked because it's challenging to equalize the pressure in the ear with the pressure in the cabin. For most people this causes mild discomfort, if anything. If you have an ear, nose or sinus infection, the best thing to do is avoid flying. If the infection is severe, you could end up with tinnitus, dizziness or even hearing loss.

Of course, unless we're talking serious infection, the business traveler has to make the best of things. Aside from checking with your doctor, who may prescribe something to help, here are some helpful tips:

TIPS FOR AVOIDING EAR BAROTRAUMA

★ Avoid alcohol because it causes the eustachian tubes to swell.

★ Stay hydrated to help the eustachian tubes function properly and to avoid irritation of nasal passages and pharynx.

★ Consult with your doctor if you've recently had ENT surgery to see if you're clear to fly.

★ Use decongestant nasal sprays or drops.

★ Make sure you're awake for landing so you can suck on a hard candy or swallow saliva to "pop" your ears.

Yawning helps too.

★ If all else fails, try inhaling through your mouth while pinching your nose closed, then exhale through your nose while it is still pinched shut. Be very careful and do this gently to avoid tearing your eardrum. As soon as one ear pops, stop.

DEEP VENOUS THROMBOSIS (BLOOD CLOTS)

If you flip to the back of any airline's inflight magazine you'll find healthy flying information, including the recommendation that you get up and move around the cabin to avoid deep venous thrombosis (DVT), a condition in which blood clots in the leg segregate and move to the lungs causing a pulmonary embolism. The clots themselves can cause a lot of pain and sometimes swelling. Once in the lungs, they present pain and difficulty breathing.

DVT is often associated with flying, yet in 2002 the Aerospace Medical Association concluded: "There is no scientific evidence of a particular link with air travel itself." This was supported by the American College of Chest Physicians in 2012: "Traveling in economy class does not increase your risk for developing a blood clot, even during long-distance travel; however, remaining immobile for long periods of time will...Long-distance travelers sitting in a window seat tend to have limited mobility, which increases their risk for DVT. This risk increases as other factors are present."

DVT is a result of sitting still for too long, which can happen in an office, car or train. In the case of airline passengers, DVT is more likely to present in people with preexisting risk factors, such as smoking, cancer, coronary artery disease, history of blood clot formation and pregnancy.

TIPS FOR AVOIDING DVT

★ Allow yourself as much leg room as possible. This is one where short people win for a change.

★ Bend and straighten your legs during the fight. Some airlines have videos you can follow. I once did Lufthansa's entire series in a coach seat without the person next to me noticing, though admittedly he was asleep.

★ Get up and walk around if it is deemed safe to do so.

★ Stay hydrated. (See Chapter 5 for tips on how to stay hydrated).

★ If you have a risk factor, talk to your doctor about compression stockings or blood thinners.

★ As much as is practical, avoid sleeping in a cramped posture or sitting in the same position for too long.

★ Avoid sleeping aids because they can cause immobility while you're asleep.

TRAVELER'S DIARRHEA

Traveler's diarrhea is the most common illness among those traveling from developed countries to developing countries. The standard advice for avoiding diarrhea is very sound: Clean your teeth with bottled water, peel fruits and vegetables, et cetera. That might work for the leisure traveler but not necessarily for the business traveler, who may be at the mercy of a host or client who determines where you're eating, what you're eating and what you're drinking.

You have the option to lock yourself in your hotel room and only come out for meetings armed with the bottled water and protein bars you brought from home, but that's not really practical. Here's the poop, sorry, I meant scoop.

The usual suspects for causing diarrhea are raw or undercooked meat, poultry, seafood, raw and unpeeled fruits and vegetables, tap water, ice, unpasteurized milk and other dairy. That doesn't leave much, does it? Food handling is hugely important because—I hate to tell you this—you usually get the trots because you've ingested fecally contaminated food or water. The risk is the same with cooked and uncooked food.

According to Traveldoctor.co.uk, "The most important determinant factor (in contracting traveler's diarrhea) is the destination of the traveler." In other words, where you are in the world makes a difference too. Latin America, Africa, the Middle East and Asia have a 50 percent rate of attack.

Be aware that you have as much chance getting traveler's

diarrhea eating street food as at a fancy restaurant. In fact, the Centers for Disease Control warn that staying at five-star hotels is worse than three or four star properties as "fancier" chefs are more likely to prepare food with bare hands!

As you travel, and your gastrointestinal tract is exposed to different organisms, your immune system might not be able to overcome these invading pathogens, so you get sick. Note that the gastrointestinal tract forms a large part of the immune system because its surface area is huge—about the size of a football field. That's a lot of ground to protect.

TOP TIPS FOR AVOIDING TRAVELER'S DIARRHEA

★ If you tend to be susceptible to gastrointestinal disorders, take as many precautions as possible. Definitely take an acidophilus supplement to keep friendly gut flora happy (these are the guys that keep "bad" bacteria at bay).

★ Trust your gut (pun intended). If a food doesn't seem right to you then it probably isn't. Use your better judgement to avoid anything that looks or smells suspicious.

★ Eat plenty of fiber to ensure that your normal, friendly gut flora stay happy and healthy.

★ Fermented foods also enhance intestinal flora. Add kombucha (my favorite—a fermented drink that makes me burp like crazy but settles my stomach faster than anything), sauerkraut or kefir to your diet; all three can be found in supermarket refrigerated sections.

★ Look for safe water. Drink bottled whenever possible and use it to clean your teeth; beware ice cubes; drink hot tea or coffee, but watch out for dodgy cream and milk.

★ Dr. Mariana Calleja recommends taking a SteriPEN with you. This is a hand-held, ultra-violet water purification system (www.steripen.com), which is handy, practical and safe for personal use.

★ Be careful with unpasteurized dairy.

★ Avoid rare-cooked meats.

★ Ask if there are any risks with local fish and seafood.

★ As much as possible, eat cooked veggies rather than salads.

★ Try to avoid fly-infested food (I've broken that one a lot).

★ Peel fruit to remove any manually transmitted germs.

★ Wash your hands just like you were brought up to do, not only after using the bathroom but also before eating.

★ Er, avoid street vendors.

★ Check out dining establishments on Trip Advisor because reviewers will often report instances of food poisoning.

★ Buffets are best avoided as you don't know how long the food has been sitting out. If this is your only option, choose cooked foods over raw.

★ Take some food with you, such as packets of miso soup or oatmeal that you can prepare yourself.

★ Have healthy prepackaged snacks handy so you don't get so hungry that you throw caution to the wind and eat the first morsel you find.

Sometimes, despite your very best efforts, you may meet a bacterium that is stronger than you. Here's what to do if that dreadful day hits.

DEALING WITH DIARRHEA

★ Hydrate with clean water. Be careful not to gulp— sip gently so your body doesn't reject it.

★ Slowly introduce plain foods such as crackers, boiled rice, broth and plain toast.

★ Avoid spicy foods.

★ Try sipping ginger tea (keep a couple of ginger tea-bags in your luggage for unexpected digestive issues). Pukka and Tazo are excellent.

★ Avoid sugary foods because sugar absorbs water from the body.

★ See if you can get Kombucha, an excellent beverage for settling the stomach. Otherwise try sparkling water or club soda.

★ Diarrhea and vomiting lead to depleted electrolytes.

Replace them with Pedialyte, if it's available, or an electrolyte supplement like Emergen-C.

★ Keep an over-the-counter remedy, such as sachets of oral rehydration salts, in your bag.

★ If you vomit more than four times in an hour, get to a doctor. You probably have food poisoning.

★ If diarrhea lasts more than a week, you have to start thinking about more serious microorganisms, such as giardia.

CONSTIPATION

Sometimes travel affects the digestive system in a completely different way, and you may find yourself constipated. The first order of the day is to drink more water to loosen up matter in the colon, and start eating more fiber. Legumes are your best friends here, along with fresh fruit and vegetables. Sometimes lack of exercise can cause constipation, too. I've found that five minutes of abdominal exercises can prompt bowel movement because they massage the internal organs.

Try the Pilates Rolling Like A Ball exercise for quick relief! Sit on a well-padded surface. If you don't have a mat, fold up a bedspread and place it on the floor. Sit with your knees bent and feet lifted, hands on your shins or behind the thighs, elbows wide. As you hold your balance here, pull your abdominals in and up. Tuck your chin, and rock back to the tips of your shoulder blades (not onto your head, please), and back up to balance. Inhale to rock back, exhale to come up. Repeat eight times.

CHAPTER 8

STRESS & RESILIENCE

Is there anything quite as destructive as stress? A leading cause of disease and sickness, of sexual dysfunction and sleeping disorders, and a brutal destroyer of psychological well-being, stress is by many accounts enemy number one.

Road warriors know stress. The world of constant traveling is a world of innumerable stressors. Well, guess what? It's about to get even worse.

While business travelers deliver a very respectable return on investment for their companies, more than justifying the expenditure on the travel itself, get ready for cost-cutting—that means more stress.

Per a 2013 review by Oxford Economics, the global forecasting venture with Oxford's business college, from 2007 to 2011, each dollar spent on business travel generated revenue of $9.50 and new profit of $2.90, and this during a recessionary period. The trend shows no sign of declining, as the same study reported that 34% of firms surveyed planned on increasing their total volume of business travel over the next few years.

> "WHILE BUSINESS TRAVELERS DELIVER A VERY RESPECTABLE RETURN ON INVESTMENT FOR THEIR COMPANIES, MORE THAN JUSTIFYING THE EXPENDITURE ON THE TRAVEL ITSELF, GET READY FOR COST-CUTTING—THAT MEANS MORE STRESS. "

But those numbers aren't benefitting road warriors. In fact, according to Global Business Travel Builds Sales and Stress, a 2014 study by Carlson Wagonlit Travel and HEC Paris, 43% of companies said they would become tougher on travel compliance policies in an attempt to reduce costs.

Tougher?!?! We're already crunched. Consider: 96% of business travelers fly in economy on domestic flights, 65% on intercontinental and 94% on continental. (Carlson Wagonlit Travel, Inc., 2012).

Now the trend is to pack customer contact into a single trip to spread transportation costs, adding days to a single trip in an effort to see more people. An already stressful vocation just got a lot more stressful.

Suffice it to say, returns on travel investment don't mention taking into account employee stress or travel fatigue. It's little surprise therefore that 64% of global business travelers surveyed by Westin Hotels and Resorts in 2014 stated that stress levels had increased over the last few years, with 30% claiming their work stress level had significantly increased over the previous year.

A 2012 study by Carlson Wagonlit Travel identified three main stressors for business travelers:

1. Lost time when it was difficult or impossible to work, creating an additional workload when they had to catch up. (This occurs when there is a poor internet connection, you're flying coach on a long-haul flight, there's no space to use a lap top or you're worried about a seat mate reading your confidential information.)

2. Surprises like losing your baggage and having to waste time shopping for replacements.

3. Disruptions, such as not being able to maintain a healthy diet or workout routine. Very early or late departure times also factor, as well as traveling on weekends, especially if you have a partner or family.

The study showed that the more travel (six to ten trips a year), the more stress. This is especially true when flying economy, using lower class hotels and traveling on weekends.

The common denominator among these stress factors is a lack of control. While frequent travelers typically are great at thinking on their feet and adapting their plans at the last minute, these particular scenarios represent the biggest challenge.

HOW STRESS WORKS:

Meanwhile, on the inside, stress initiates physiological processes that can have long-term health implications.

When you get stressed, your body sends out adrenaline in the form of epinephrine whose job it is to tell your body to go into fight-or-flight mode, as if you are being chased by a lion. Meanwhile, the liver releases glucose from its glycogen stores so you can reap the energy and run as fast as your legs will carry you.

Once out of harm's way, you would switch into rest mode, and glucose release would return to normal. But if you're constantly stressed, like many people nowadays, you're going to keep releasing glucose, which raises blood sugar levels. This sustained activity can lead to insulin resistance and diabetes, to mention only a few serious results of stress.

When most people learn how dangerous stress is, they find they have yet another thing to stress out about. But *Mile High and Healthy* travelers can take advantage of stress relievers.

GETTING RID OF STRESS BY BUILDING RESILIENCE:

Resilience is a buzzword in stress management these days, and rightly so. Resilience is the human capacity to get through stress, catastrophe and adversity, as manifested at an extreme level when people recover in the aftermath of tornedoes and hurricanes.

Having resilience doesn't mean you won't encounter

difficult situations. It's about how you handle and work through them. Resilient people tend to bounce back from adversity. They don't experience less trauma, but they're able to recuperate faster.

You don't have to be born with resilience. You can develop resilience by taking small steps to create habits that will help you prepare for and face challenging circumstances. The first step to any change is to take a step back mentally and reflect on a situation. Humans (and therefore companies) tend to stay stuck in habitual patterns, repeating them because that's how things have always been done or because of significant investments of time or money. This is known as the "sunk cost bias", and it is why there's pressure to keep going even if the results aren't what was wanted.

> "...BUSINESS TRAVELERS WITH MULTIPLE AGENDAS ARE PRONE TO MUDDLED THINKING AND POOR DECISION MAKING BECAUSE THEY ARE JUGGLING SO MANY BALLS AT ONCE. IN OTHER WORDS, MULTI-TASKING IS OUT."

When it comes to how we take care of ourselves, this means potentially running yourself into the ground. But by stepping back and taking stock, you can see the big picture better, think more clearly and, ultimately, perform better. Ironically, travel provides the perfect opportunity for this. As you're usually on your own on a plane, in a car or hotel room, take the time to step off the hamster wheel and ask yourself some big-picture questions.

Tailor your questions to your physical and psychological resilience goals. Physical resilience might include improving your diet, exercising more and finding time for rest and relaxation. Psychological resilience might be examining your beliefs about a real or hypothetical situation.

What is your go-to internal chatter when faced with a stressful situation? Stress often starts with unconscious beliefs, but there is nothing to stop you from creating new beliefs. How do you want to behave next time your flight is delayed five hours? What beliefs do you want to establish so you're not stressed out next time this happens?

Once you have established your goal, break it down into small, manageable steps. It is easier to create new habits that way, rather than thinking you have to take a massive leap to establish a new behavioral pattern. "Tiny changes can be profoundly good. People assume an all-or-nothing approach. You either have this busy life or you're farming goats somewhere and eating muesli. They don't see that small adjustments can make a big difference," says Averil Leimon, a psychologist who is co-author of *Positive Psychology For Dummies* and one of the UK's top 10 coaches according to *The Independent*.

Positive small changes might include adding one glass of water to your daily intake, taking a 15-minute walk every day, getting away from your desk and stretching every 90 minutes. Look for opportunities to apply resilience in your daily routine.

AVERIL LEIMON'S TIPS FOR BUILDING RESILIENCE

Accept the setback. Know that setbacks happen to everyone. And realize that you may never understand what happened.

Face your fears. It's normal to feel insecure, but don't cower and avoid uncertainty.

Be patient. Reflect and think about what you plan to do, but don't rush—it will only aggravate the process.

Go beyond your comfort zone. Take risks. Go after that job you think you can't do. Doing so will build self-esteem and resilience.

Find your hero. Think about people who have survived adversity, like Christopher Reeve or Oprah. Use them as your role models.

Know what you want. If you have goals it's easier to make plans and move forward.

Be a problem-solver. Don't be the victim. Instead, learn to be proactive.

One step at a time. To move forward, the enormity of the task (such as finding a new job after a lay-off) may seem insurmountable. Focus on each step you must take, not the entire undertaking.

Seek support. Talk to friends, family or a therapist.

Be kind to yourself. Disappointments are a source of stress, so exercise, eat right and get rest.

Business travelers tend to be rather heroic about stress

"I've visited six countries in the last three days and only had nine hours of sleep" is the kind of bragging we road warriors have earned the hard way, treating terrible conditions as a badge of honor rather than a cause for concern. This in itself can be a way of coping with an inadequate travel policy or unrealistic expectations from management. But in the long run, that attitude will result in failure.

Being cavalier can lead to a severe case of "presenteeism" where you're showing up and going through the motions, but not performing well. Let's say you have to travel on the weekend then go straight to work the following Monday. If you're not fully rested, you'll run on auto-pilot, appearing to be present but not really working at your best capacity. Travelers often don't realize how deeply exhausted they really are.

Presenteeism generates extra work in the long run. Say you work on a report during an overnight flight because you feel you "should," but you're tired. On revisiting your work the next day, you see errors and inaccuracies. You have to re-do it. In reality, you've gone through the motions of doing the report, which makes you feel less anxious for a while, and yet it generates more stress by wasting the time it takes you to redo it. Ask yourself, what is the worst that can happen if you take time off to recharge your batteries?

Leimon is adamant: "Signs and symptoms of stress are not inevitable. We choose to do or not to do stress." Arm yourself with some of the coping mechanisms below so you can learn not to elect stress.

TIPS FOR QUICK DE-STRESSING:

BREATHE. Controlling your breathing is the fastest way to counter stress. It's free, it's simple and you can do it absolutely anywhere. Inhaling and exhaling slowly calms the sympathetic nervous system. Start by inhaling to a count of five and then exhaling to a count of five. Do this for about one minute. Eventually, adjust your breathing until you're taking a big inhalation for one count and exhaling for nine counts. Build up to this gradually.

CARVE OUT SOME "ME" TIME. You have the opportunity to take time for yourself whether it's to meditate, exercise or simply clear your head. If you have trouble prioritizing for yourself, schedule your alone time like you would any other appointment and stick to it.

TAKE BREAKS EVERY 90 MINUTES. Even if it's just taking a moment to step away from your desk and change your environment, break out of your routine. You'll come back refreshed. I take a 15-minute exercise break every 90 minutes when I'm working from my home office. Stepping away from my desk clears my head, making room for ideas and inspiration that I can take back to my work. I've learned to keep a voice recorder handy so I don't forget my pearls of wisdom.

TAKE YOUR VACATION. The stats are scary. According to the US Travel Association, Americans fail to use 429 million vacation days every year. That's $54 billion in earned benefits lost by forfeiting vacations. In essence, it's like working for free if you don't take your vacation days.

JOURNAL. If stress is manifesting frequently in your life, it might be helpful to journal how you feel so you can recognize the triggers and patterns. First thing in the morning is the best time for this as you still have access to the unconscious thoughts that will be gone once you're fully awake. In *The Artist's Way: A Spiritual Path To Higher Creativity*, Julia Cameron recommends keeping your journal by your bed and reaching for it while you are still half-asleep. By writing first thing, you have the chance to "brain dump" the repressed thoughts that are bothering you, getting them out of your head, as it were, and leaving you free to move through your day without them.

GET A SUPPORT TEAM. Surround yourself with friends and family who believe in your strengths and abilities. If you prefer objective support, a life coach or therapist can help.

MEDITATE. I resisted meditation for years on the grounds that it was too woo-woo, and I didn't have time for it. Enter Graham Doke, an ex-City of London lawyer and investment banker, who left his extremely successful career to study Eastern philosophy and Eastern and Western psychology, combining these disciplines with modern neuroscience and physics.

Doke explained how business travelers with multiple agendas are prone to muddled thinking and poor decision-making because they are juggling so many balls at once. In other words, multitasking is out. With mind training, or meditation, you can clear the mental clutter, learn to focus, and make better, more profitable decisions.

If you're a meditation neophyte, I recommend the Anamaya app (www.anamaya.co.). Doke was the principal architect of this app, which takes you through the process of learning how to meditate then gradually progresses through different levels. It's also the perfect solution for what I call "finding space in a crowded place." You can listen to it on a plane, on a train or in an airport to escape from the hubbub around you.

CREATE A SELF-CARE MENU. This is a list of things you really like to do to relax. It's very personal and specific to you. Activities may include taking a bubble bath, calling a friend for 15 minutes, pottering around your garden, listening to music, dancing around your living room, having a nap, reading cartoons or curling up with a good book.

Pick one item per day, and schedule it as if you have to. You'll soon get into the routine of doing something just for yourself every day. Having a self-care menu is a valuable tool against self-medication with alcohol or food during times of stress.

> "TINY CHANGES CAN BE PROFOUNDLY GOOD. PEOPLE ASSUME AN ALL OR NOTHING APPROACH. YOU EITHER HAVE THIS BUSY LIFE OR YOU'RE FARMING GOATS SOMEWHERE AND EATING MUESLI. THEY DON'T SEE THAT SMALL ADJUSTMENTS CAN MAKE A BIG DIFFERENCE," SAYS AVERIL LEIMON, AUTHOR OF *POSITIVE PSYCHOLOGY FOR DUMMIES.*

BE BAD. Frequent travelers are usually A types, programmed for perfection. Everything has to be right, and you have to be good at everything. But once in a while it's good to be bad, to do something naughty or out of your usual pattern. Thomas Leonard, considered the father of life coaching, explained it like this: "People are not perfect, and we shouldn't pretend to be. In a way it is inauthentic to live life pretending to be so perfect. That is the real lack of integrity."

Please don't go and rob a bank on the grounds that I told you to do something bad, but anything else that feels like something you probably shouldn't do would work. Maybe

> "PICK QUALITY OVER QUANTITY. OVERCOMMITTING LEADS TO BEING OVERWHELMED, AND THE FIRST PERSON TO SUFFER IS YOU. WHEN YOU LEARN TO SAY NO, YOU CAN SCHEDULE SOME OF THAT TIME FOR YOURSELF."

you'll power off all your devices for half an hour, or stop being reactive to emails (62% of business travelers feel the need to read an email as soon as it arrives, according to a 2005 study in the *International Journal of Human Resources Development and Management*) or play hooky and go see a movie. Pick something on your to-do list to consciously not do!

Being bad puts you in charge of your life rather than letting an inherent belief system take over. And it can feel so darned good.

LEARN TO SAY "NO." You have to discipline yourself to say no to unwanted or unnecessary engagements. Sometimes you might feel pressure to attend every single business engagement to which you're invited so that you look like a team player. Pick quality over quantity. Overcommitting leads to being overwhelmed, and the first person to suffer is you. When you learn to say no, you can schedule some of that time for yourself.

10 GREAT AIRPORT
HANGOUTS FOR DE-STRESSING

Having trouble scheduling "me" time? Then take advantage of being in an airport. You don't have to work or sit at the bar. Many airports have fabulous opportunities for chilling out, including spas, shopping and exercise facilities (see Chapter 3).

Have a treatment. XpresSpa is now at 56 airports worldwide and offers massage, nail care and skin care. See xpresspa.com for locations. Enjoy reflexology at Singapore's Changi Airport, or jet lag recovery and Thai massages at Bangkok Suvarnabhumi Airport's Spa Centre.

Meditate. Albuquerque International Sunport and Raleigh-Durham International Airport provide meditation areas.

Play pool. Rack 'em up! Both pool and billiards are available at Dubai International's Terminal C.

Visit the aquarium. An aquarium at an airport? Yes, indeed—at San Francisco International Airport.

Watch a movie. You can do it in style at Hong Kong International Airport's IMAX theater, or visit the iSports area with simulators for soccer, basketball, golf, boxing, skiing, car racing and shooting.

View some art. You'll find galleries and exhibits at Miami International, Amsterdam's Schipol (even boasts a

Rembrandt), Denver, Edinburgh (contemporary Scottish art for purchase), Hartsfield-Jackson Atlanta, Philadelphia International, Ottawa, Los Angeles, San Francisco, Sacramento and Heathrow, Terminal 5.

Take a nap. Sleeping pods are the latest innovation to help passengers disengage from the mêlée of the concourse. You'll find sleeping pods in Abu Dhabi, Dubai and Helsinki airports (gosleep.areo). More elaborate variations can be found at Sheremetyevo International Airport, Munich, New Delhi, Heathrow (Terminal 4) and London Gatwick (South Terminal). You can rent a room by the hour (not as dodgy as it sounds) in Dallas through MinuteSuites if you want to nap, work or just hang out in peace and quiet. Sleepinginairports.com rates airports for their facilities.

Visit a butterfly garden. Changi Airport, Singapore, boasts a two-story butterfly grotto, 27-foot waterfall and a Balinese rooftop pool.

Take a city tour. Passengers with a minimum five-and-a-half-hour layover at Changi can take a free two-and-a-half-hour bus tour of the city. The Heritage Tour runs four times daily, and the City Lights Tour runs twice daily. There's a Left Luggage facility for your carry-on bags.

Perfect your swing. Golf via a 300m driving range, 18-hole putting course and a "swing analysis center" at Golf Town, Incheon Airport Seoul.

SECURITY AND ANXIETY

Stress can be caused on a very visceral level by anxiety regarding personal safety. Employees tend to be uncomfortable sharing their travel-related anxieties, yet many find themselves sleeping with one eye or ear open because they don't feel safe in their hotel room. Employers have a legal obligation to provide an adequate care of duty while you're on the road, but here are some steps you can take to protect yourself.

If travel policy permits, ensure that your flight arrives during daylight hours.

Carolyn Pearson, founder of Maiden-voyage.com, the networking site for female business travelers, recommends that if you're arriving in an unfamiliar city, country or territory, look at the route between the airport and your destination on Google Streetview so you can be sure you are being taken in the right direction.

> "IF TRAVELING TO A DESTINATION WITH A DIFFERENT ALPHABET, SEE IF YOU CAN GET YOUR DESTINATION CITY AND HOTEL IN THE LOCAL SCRIPT ON YOUR LUGGAGE LABELS. THERE ARE PLENTY OF WEBSITES THAT WILL FACILITATE THIS."

I happen to have a degree in Arabic which makes me a bit geeky about other alphabets and scripts. If traveling to a destination with a different alphabet, see if you can get your destination city and hotel in the local script on your luggage labels. There are plenty of websites that will facilitate this.

Security issues apply to both male and female travelers, according to Pearson. Women may or may not be intrinsically programmed to limit how much personal information they give away about themselves when talking in public, but—at the end of the day—drugs can be added to anyone's drink, so don't keep yours unattended.

At the hotel, whether you're male or female, if your room number is announced out loud on checking in, ask for a different room and for the number to be conveyed to you discreetly. Two weeks before writing this paragraph, I checked into a well-known hotel in a major European city. My room number was announced loud and clear in front of the two strangers also at the check-in desk. Thieves don't discriminate by gender.

As a firefighter's daughter, I also recommend keeping your room on the sixth floor or lower if you're worried about tackling the fire escape—anything higher and your floor might not be reachable by ladders. And, if you really want to listen to my dad's advice, walk the hotel floor corridor when you arrive and count the doors to the nearest fire exit. If you fancy some cardio, take the stairs to make sure the exit door isn't bolted shut (my pet hate when I'm trying to get some exercise without hitting the gym).

RELATIONSHIPS

A survey by Westin Hotels and Resorts in 2014 stated: "Priorities between work and personal life are one of the biggest barriers to well-being for 54% of global business travelers."

An earlier Carlson Wagonlit Travel survey from 2012 showed much the same thing. Travelers experienced increased amounts of stress when they had a wife, husband or partner and when they had children, particularly when traveling on weekends and stays of more than three nights.

Some think that relationship issues should be easier to handle from the road these days thanks to Skype, FaceTime and unlimited mobile phone plans. But technology, while valuable, isn't always the answer.

A couple of years ago, I was working in a hotel room and heard shouting from the next room, a man yelling at his partner (I assumed) on the other end of the phone. "Don't you realize that I'm here working on a f***ing million-dollar deal and all I get from you is grief. F*** off and find somebody else. I don't want to hear it right now."

He repeated the scenario the next morning. Not the best way to use one's unlimited phone plan, evidently.

Here are seven strategies to keep the flame kindled, and to let sanity and order reign, so that the course of true love can run smoothly whether you're five feet or five thousand miles apart.

Not taking each other for granted seems clichéd but, as I like to say, clichés are clichés for a reason. If complacency occurs in the course of "normal" relationships, imagine how extreme it may become when one party is away much of the time. While you're absent, the house is managed; bills are paid; chores are completed; and the kids and pets are fed and watered, all this while your partner may be working full time. Even if the help is farmed out, that still has to be arranged and supervised. A little "thank you" here and there will go a long way. An "I appreciate you" will go even further.

Be honest about how you're coping with the separation rather than holding back how you really feel. The road warrior persona is a toughie. You have to be alert, adaptable and street-smart. And did I mention really good at your job while dealing with the stressors that frequent travel can deliver? When it's time for your Skype session, put the tough nut aside and let your vulnerability shine.

Plan special time for your return well in advance rather than arriving home with vague intentions of "doing something special." This one is key, because after a long business trip, you'll walk in the door too tired to plan anything. So plan it in advance. That way you both have something to look forward to outside of the daily grind. Focus on the details of your romantic interlude. Paint a picture of it in your mind's eye. It will keep you going through a boring meeting!

Do things together while you're away. If you're in the same time zone, keep the Skype or the phone on and watch a favourite TV show together, or just be. If you're not in the same time zone, a wake-up call from the partner that is ahead in time can be a lovely start to the day.

Show your loved one that you are thinking of them while you're away. Buying presents last minute at the airport doesn't count, but buying something spontaneously because you know they'd like it or because it reminds you of them speaks volumes. Gifts aren't necessary every trip, but thoughtfulness is.

Be sure that your partner doesn't avoid addressing problems because you're away, and they don't want to trouble you. If you were coming home every night, you'd have to deal with the issues and still go to work the next day. Address matters as they arrive rather than leaving them to accumulate. That way you can both move on.

Be sensitive to adjusting when returning home. Maybe you're returning from your trip brimming with excitement about the latest deal or great meeting. Meanwhile, your partner who has stayed home looking after the kids and has been dealing with seeming disasters and going to work every day doesn't care if you've been to Barbados or Bangor. Conversely, you arrive jet lagged and drained while your loved one is bursting with energy on seeing you. Set parameters for at least 15 minutes of alone time so you can regroup in your own milieu, even if you've been alone on the road. It's time to reset the odometer, and that might mean locking the bathroom door.

> "MEANWHILE, YOUR PARTNER WHO HAS STAYED HOME LOOKING AFTER THE KIDS AND HAS BEEN DEALING WITH SEEMING DISASTERS AND GOING TO WORK EVERY DAY, DOESN'T CARE IF YOU'VE BEEN TO BARBADOS OR BANGOR."

EPILOGUE

I've run three culinary and Pilates retreats in Italy's Piedmont. The owner of the fabulous host property always observed, "Americans show up with bags full of nutrition bars but then they never eat them." Thank goodness for that.

While much of my travel is for work, the real motivator for me is the chance to eat and drink my way through any culture. How can you go to Italy and eschew pasta and bread in favor of a protein bar?

You can stay healthy and well while still tasting your way across the globe. Take the time to explore the culinary and oenological opportunities that are presented while practicing the tips you've learned from this book. You see, it's not that there's travel and there's staying healthy, they can meld.

The path to wellness is its own journey. You can handle that. You're a traveler.

SOURCES

Chapter 1: Healthy Eating

"Carotenoid bioavailability is higher from salads ingested with full-fat than with fat reduced salad dressings as measured with electrochemical detection." *American Journal of Clinical Nutrition*, August 2004.

Craig WJ, Mangels AR. "Position of the American Dietetic Association: vegetarian diets." *Journal American Dietetic Association*. 2009; 109:1266-1282.

Young LR, Nestle M. "The contribution of expanding portion sizes to the US obesity epidemic." *American Journal of Public Health,* 2002 Feb;92(2):246-9.

Michael Pollan, Food Revolution Summit, April 25, 2015.

http://www.qsrmagazine.com/outside-insights/fly-high-airport-concessions

http://www.usatoday.com/story/travel/flights/2013/08/04/airports-food-trucks/2609067/

http://www.pcrm.org/health/reports/2014-airport-food-review

http://www.flychicago.com/OHare/EN/AboutUs/Sustainability/Aeroponic-Garden.aspx

http://www.upenn.edu/pennnews/news/smaller-portions-restaurants-and-markets-may-explain-french-paradox-rich-foods-and-svelte-popul

http://www.marketwatch.com/story/7-disappearing-hotel-amenities-2014-01-08

Chapters 2 and 3: Exercise

McGill SM, Brown S. "Creep Response of the lumbar spine to prolonged flexion." *Clinical Biomechanics* 1992; 7:43-46.

Black A, Katia M, Lorn A, Narden H, Margareta: "Association between sitting and occupational lower back pain." *European Spine Journal, Springer-Verlag* 007-02-01. http://dx.doi.org/10.1007/s00586-006-0143-7.

McKenzie R, May S. "These tissues may become susceptible to fatigue failure, and the insidious development of musculoskeletal symptoms despite no obvious trauma," *The Lumbar Spine Mechanical Diagnosis and Therapy,* 2003;2nd ed.Waikanae, New Zealand: Spinal Publications, New Zealand. p. 103-120.

Mi-Yong Lee, Hae-Yong Lee, Min-Sik Yong: "Characteristics of Cervical Position Sense in Subjects with Forward Head Posture." *Journal of Physical Therapy Science*, Nov. Vol 26 (2014), No. 11.

Burgess-Limerick R, Ployy A, Ankrum DR: "The effect of imposed and self-selected computer monitor height on posture and gaze angle." *Clinical Biomechanics*, 1998 Dec;13(8):584-592.

http://businesstravel.about.com/od/healthsafety/a/Preventing-Pain.htm

http://www.backsafe.com/newsletters/pdfs/laptop.pdf

http://www.telegraph.co.uk/news/health/expat-health/8373174/Long-haul-flights-can-be-a-real-pain-in-the-back.html

http://www.nytimes.com/2004/01/06/business/business-travel-a-long-trip-a-crammed-flight-and-a-lingering-pain.html?pagewanted=1

http://www.wsj.com/articles/SB122938297526708695 (When Your Laptop Is A Big Pain in the Neck)

"THE WEARABLES REPORT: Growth trends, consumer attitudes, and why smartwatches will dominate," *Business Insider*, May 2015

The 49 Best Health and Fitness Apps of 2015, http://greatlist.com/fitness/best-health-fitness-apps

Wearable Tech Device Awareness Surpasses 50% - npd.com. https://www.npd.com/wps/portal/npd/us/news/press-releases/wearable-tech-device-awareness-surpasses-50-percent-among-us-consumers-according-to-npd/

Best Fitness Trackers for 2015, pcmag.com http://www.pcmag.com/article2/0,2817,2404445,00.asp

www.yogatraveltree.com
www.dfwairport.com

www.flychicago.com

www.burlingtonintlairport.com

http://www.finavia.fi/en/helsinki-airport/

www.changiairport.com

www.yvr.ca

www.schipol.nl

Chapter 4: Energy

Hoppe C, et al. "High intakes of milk, but not meat, increase insulin and insulin resistance in 8 year old boys." *European Journal of Clinical Nutrition*, 2005; 59:393-8.

Liljeberg EH, Bjorck I. "Milk as a supplement to mixed meals may elevate postprandial insulinanemia." *European Journal of Clinical Nutrition*, 2001;55:994-999.

Heany RP. "Effects of caffeine on bone and the calcium economy." *Food And Chemical Toxicology*; 2002 Sep;40(9):1263-70.

Boekema PJ, Samsom M, van Berge Henegouwen GP, Smout AJ. "Coffee and gastrointestinal function: facts and fiction. A review." *Scandinavian Journal of Gastroenterology Supplement*. 1999;230:35-9.

Lovallo, William R. PhD; Whitsett, Thomas L. MD; al'Absi, Mustafa PhD; Sung, Bong Hee PhD; Vincent, Andrea S. PhD; Wilson, Michael F. MD ."Caffeine Stimulation of Cortisol Secretion Across the Waking Hours in Relation to Caffeine Intake Levels." *Psychosomatic Medicine*,September/October 2005 - Volume 67 - Issue 5 - pp 734-739.

Verhoef P, Pasman WJ, Trinette van Vliet, Rob Urgert, and Martijn B Katan. "Contribution of caffeine to the homocysteine-raising effect of coffee: a randomized controlled trial in humans1[2,3]" *The American Journal of Clinical Nutrition*, December 2002 vol. 76 no. 6 1244-1248.

Akimoto K, Inamori M, Iida H, Endo H, Akiyama T, Ikeda T, Fujita K, Takahashi H, Yoneda M, Goto A, Abe Y, Kobayashi N, Kirikoshi H, Kubota K, Saito S, Nakajima A. "Does postprandial coffee intake enhance gastric emptying?: a crossover study using continuous real time 13C breath test (BreathID system). " *Hepatogastroenterology*, 2009 May-Jun;56(91-92):918-20.

Hazum E, Sabatka JJ, Chang KJ, Brent DA, Findlay JW, Cuatrecasas P. "Morphine in cow and human milk: could dietary morphine constitute a ligand for specific morphine (mu) receptors?" *Science*, 1981 Aug 28;213(4511):1010-2.

Teschemacher H, Koch G, Brantl V. "Milk protein-derived opioid receptor ligands." *Biopolymers*. 1997;43(2):99-117.

Aslam M, Hurley WL. "Biological Activities of Peptides Derived from Milk Proteins." University of Illinois Extension http://livestocktrail.illinois.edu/dairynet/paperDisplay.cfm?ContentID=249

http://www.health.harvard.edu/healthy-eating/glycemic_index_and_glycemic_load_for_100_foods

Chapter 5: Jet Lag and Jet Stress

Herxheimer A, Petrie KJ. "Melatonin for the prevention and treatment of jet lag." *Cochrane Review*, Issue 4.

Waterhouse J, Reilly T, Atkinson G, Edwards B. "Jet lag: trends and coping strategies." *The Lancet*. 2007 Mar 31;369(9567):1117–29.

Oschman JL. "Can Electrons Act As Antioxidants? A Review and Commentary." *Journal of Alternative and Complementary Medicine*, 2007 Nov; 13(9):955-67

Chevalier G, Sinatra S, Oschman J, Sokal K, Sokal P. "Earthing: Health Implications of Reconnecting the Human Body to the Earth's Surface Electrons." *Journal of Environmental and Public Health*. 2012; 2012:291541.

Sokal K, Sokal P. "Earthing The Human Body Influences Physiologic Processes." *Journal of Alternative and Complementary Medicine*. 2011 Apr; 17(4):301-8.

Ghaly M and Taplitz D. "The biological effects of grounding the human body during sleep as measured by cortisol levels and subjective reporting of sleep, pain and stress." *Journal of Alternative and Complementary Medicine*, 2004; 10(5): 767-776.

Forbes-Robertson, S.; Dudley, E.; Vadgama, P.; Cook, C.; Drawer, S.; Kilduff, L. (2012). "Circadian Disruption and Remedial Interventions". *Sports Medicine* 42 (3): 185–208.

Bagshaw M, DeVoll JR, Jennings RT, McCrary BF, Northrup SE, Rayman RB, et al. Medical Guidelines for Airline Passengers. Alexandria, VA: Aerospace Medical Association; 2002 [cited 2012 Sep 26].

T. L. Leise & M. E. Harrington & P. C. Molyneux & I. Song & H. Queenan & E. Zimmerman & G. S. Lall & S. M. Biello. "Voluntary exercise can strengthen the circadian system in aged mice." *Age*, 2013 Dec;35(6):2137-52. doi: 10.1007/s11357-012-9502-y. Epub 2013 Jan 23.

Reilly, T. (1998). "Travel: Physiology, jet-lag, strategies." *Encyclopedia of Sports Medicine and Science*, T.D. Fahey (Editor). Internet Society for Sport Science. 12 July 1998. www.sportsci.org/encyc/jetlag/jetlag.html

Bunnell DE, Agnew JW, Horvath SM, Jopson L, Wills M. "Passive body heating and sleep: influence of proximity to sleep." Institute of Environmental Stress, University of California, Santa Barbara.

Chavalier G. "The Earth's Electrical Surface Potential: A summary of present understanding," January 2007, California Institute for Human Science, Graduate School & Research Center, Encinitas, CA

"Aeromedical Requirements for Dehydration – Do You Know The Answer?" Nina Anderson, Corporate Pilot and Author of "Eliminating Pilot Error."

"The Need For Broad Spectrum Trace Minerals In Aerospace Environments." White Paper by Nina Anderson, Corporate Pilot and Author of "Eliminating Pilot Error."

Ober C, Sinatra S, Zucker, M. "Earthing: The Most Important Health Discovery Ever?" Basic Health Publications, 2010.

"Electrolytes, The Spark of Life," Gillian Martlew, ND. Nature's Publishing Limited, 1994.

http://www.flinders.edu.au/sabs/psychology/research/labs/sleep/bas.cfm

http://wwwnc.cdc.gov/travel/yellowbook/2014/chapter-2-the-pre-travel-consultation/jet-lag

http://wwwnc.cdc.gov/travel/yellowbook/2014/chapter-6-conveyance-and-transportation-issues/air-travel

www.earthinginstitute.net

Chapter 6: Sleep

Johns NP, Johns J, Porasuphatana S, Plaimee P, Sae-Teaw M. "Dietary intake of melatonin from tropical fruit altered urinary excretion of 6-sulfatoxymelatonin in healthy volunteers". Journal of Agricultural and Food Chemistry, 2013 Jan 30;61(4):913-9.

Howatson G, Bell PG, Tallent J, Middleton B, McHugh MP, Ellis J. "Effect of tart cherry juice (Prunus cerasus) on melatonin levels and enhanced sleep quality." *European Journal of Nutrition.* 2012 Dec;51(8):909-16.

Realnatural News. Research Confirms Tart Cherries Help Sleep Quality and Duration. http://www.realnatural.org/research-confirms-tart-cherries-help-sleep-quality/

Bunnell DE, Agnew JW, Horvath SM, Jopson L, Wills M. "Passive body heating and sleep: influence of proximity to sleep." Institute of Environmental Stress, University of California, Santa Barbara.

Knutson KL, Spiegel K, Penev P, Van Cauter E. "The Metabolic Consequences of Sleep Deprivation." *Sleep Medicine Review.* 2007 Jun; 11(3): 163–178. Published online 2007 Apr. doi: 10.1016/j.smrv.2007.01.002.

Speigel K, Leproult R, Van Cauter E. "Impact of sleep debt on metabolic and endocrine function." *The Lancet,* 1999 Oct 23;354(9188):1435-9.

Arendt J, Skene DJ. "Melatonin as a chronobiotic." *Sleep MedIcine Review.* 2005 Feb;9(1):25-39.

Chan JK, Trinder J, Colrain IM, Nicholas CL. "The acute effects of alcohol on sleep electroencephalogram power spectra in late adolescence." *Alcoholism Clinical and Experimental Research*, 2015 Feb;39(2):291-9. doi: 10.1111/acer.12621. Epub 2015 Jan 16.

Youngstedt SD. "Effects of Exercise on Sleep." *Clinics in Sports Medicine*, April 2005, Volume 24, Issue 2, pages 355-365.

Ferrell JM, Chiang JYL. "Circadian rhythms in liver metabolism and disease." *Acta Pharmaceutica Sinica B*, Chinese Pharmaceutical Association, Institute of Materia Medica, Chinese Academy of Medical Sciences. January 2015.

http://sleepfoundation.org/media-center/press-release/annual-sleep-america-poll-exploring-connections-communications-technology-use- 2011 Sleep In America Poll, National Sleep Foundation

Chapter 7: How to Avoid Getting Sick on the Road

Bagshaw M, Nicolls DN. "The aircraft cabin environment." In: Keystone JS, Freedman DO, Kozarsky PE, Connor BA, Nothdurft HO, editors. *Travel Medicine*. 3rd ed. Philadelphia: Saunders Elsevier; 2013. p. 405–12.

Racette SB, Spearie CA, Phillips KM, Lin X, Ma L, Ostlund R. "Phytosterol-deficient and high-phytosterol diets developed for controlled feeding studies." Journal of the American Dietetic Association, 2009. Dec: 109 (12): 2043-2051.

Penttinen-Damdimopoulou PE, Power KA, Hurmerinta TT, Nurmi T, Van der Saag PT, Mäkelä S. "Dietary sources of lignans and isoflavones modulate responses to estradiol in estrogen reporter mice." *Molecular Nutrition and Food Research.*

Olson JA. "Needs and sources of carotenoids and vitamin A."*Nutrition Reviews*, 1994 - nutritionreviews.oxfordjournals.org

"New DVT Guidelines: No Evidence to Support Economy Class Syndrome. Oral Contraceptives, Sitting in a Window Seat, Advanced Age, and Pregnancy Increase DVT Risk in Long-distance Travelers" February 7, 2012. *CHEST*, American College of Chest Physicians.

Hocking MB, Foster HD. "Common cold transmission in commercial aircraft: Industry and passenger implications." *Volume:3 Issue:1 Journal of Environmental Health Review, 2004.*

Zitter J, Mazonson P, Miller D, Hulley S, Balmes J. "Aircraft cabin air recirculation and symptoms of the common cold." *Journal of the American Medical Association*2002, 288, 483-486.

Barry P, Mason N, O'Callaghan C "Nasal mucociliary transport is impaired at altitude". *European Respiratory Journal,* 1997 10: 35-37.

Abubakar I. "Tuberculosis and air travel: a systematic review and analysis of policy." The Lancet Infectious Diseases, 2010 Mar;10(3):176-83. doi: 10.1016/S1473-3099(10)70028-1.

http://www.health.harvard.edu/staying-healthy/how-to-boost-your-immune-system

Mayo Clinic. Airplane ear: definition. Rochester, MN: Mayo Clinic; 2010 [cited 2012 Sep 26]. Available from :http://www.mayoclinic.com/health/airplane-ear/DS00472.

www.dietaryfiberfood.com

http://www.asma.org/asma/media/asma/Travel-Publications/paxguidelines.pdf

Chapter 8: Stress & Resilience

J. Stricker et al., "Risk factors for psychological stress among international business travelers," *Occupational and Environmental Medicine,* 56:245-252 (1999).

Stress Triggers for Business Travelers Traveler Survey Analysis, Carlson Wagonlit Travel, 2012.

AirPlus Traveller Productivity. "How to tailor your travel policy to improve traveler performance." AirPlus International, 2012.

Segalla, Michael. "An international study of dysfunctional e-mail usage and attitudes among managers." *International Journal of Human Resources Development and Management,* 2005.

Global Well-being Survey, Westin Hotels & Resorts, 2014.

Oxford Economics 2013, "The Role of Business Travel in the US Economic Recovery." US Travel Association, NY, 2013.

Segalla M, Ciobanu C, Rouzies D, Lebunetel V. "Global Business Travel Builds Sales and Stress," Carlson Wagonlit Travel and HEC (Ecole des Hautes Etudes Commerciales de Paris). April 2014.

https://maidenvoyagedotcom.wordpress.com/2015/01/31/7-tips-to-keep-your-relationship-grounded-while-youre-on-the-road-by-jayne-mcallister/

http://skift.com/2015/06/08/skift-survey-majority-of-americans-will-take-little-to-no-vacation-this-summer/

http://www.projecttimeoff.com/resources/fact-sheets/us-travel-time-case-study

Further Reading

Breaking the Food Seduction: The Hidden Reasons Behind Food Cravings – and 7 Steps to End Them Naturally, Neal Barnard

Farewell Jet Lag, Cures from a Flight Attendant, Christopher Babayode

Food and Healing, How What You Eat Determines Your Health, Your Well-Being, and the Quality of Your Life," Annemarie Colbin

Mindless Eating: Why We Eat More Than We Think, Brian Wansink

Nourishing Wisdom, Marc David

Sick and Tired: Reclaim Your Inner Terrain, Robert O. Young

The Artist's Way: A Spiritual Path to Higher Creativity, Julia Cameron

The Blood Sugar Solution: The UltraHealthy Program for Losing Weight, Preventing Disease and Feeling Great Now, Mark Hyman

The China Study: Startling Implications For Diet, Weight Loss and Long-term Health, T. Colin Campbell

"Travel Healthy: A Road Warrior's Guide to Eating Healthy, Natasha Léger

Sleep: A Very Short Introduction, Steven W. Lockley and Russell G. Foster

ACKNOWLEDGEMENTS

To Granddad Keyburn, for giving me the travel bug, and to Grandma, for teaching me how to eat real food on the go.

To my family, who tolerated my "presenteeism" when I came to visit them in the UK but spent all my time writing this book. Dad and Sue, Mum and Chris, Hilda and Jack—next time I visit we'll actually have to socialize. To Michael McAllister, for feeding me and dealing with my unwashed self as I sat (with perfect posture, of course) glued to my computer for weeks on end.

To my Scouse cousins, Nicola Billington, the very first person to read this manuscript, and Chris Billington, for telling me to go big or go home. Since April 2015, I do so in his memory. *You'll Never Walk Alone.*

To Bob Morris and the Story Farm team. I'm so glad that a friendship with Bob sparked many years ago has translated into this project. While I cowered at the mere thought of an editor, Scott Morris and Veronica Randall were the most wonderful and encouraging taskmasters. Given my penchant for hyphens, Anglicisms and medieval language, they deserve canonization.

To James Agnew, MD, PhD, Anatomy and Physiology teacher extraordinaire. Thank you for your infinite patience and for making sure I got all the science right. And for sharing your own amazing travel stories!

To Cher Murphy, the best publicist ever, who follows her calling with such joy and generosity of spirit.

To Susan Parker, for making me show up for myself when I

really didn't want to.

To Justin Kidd, for compiling research that would have taken me hours, and completing it quickly, efficiently and accurately. And, best of all, presenting it to me in a format that I could read and understand.

Thanks to Kirk Cheyfitz, for telling me to write a book; for being the best boss ever; for telling me to voice my ideas; and for sponsoring my green card. I would literally not be where I am if it weren't for you.

To Gina McDonald and Carina Dingemans, for countless hours on different continents enjoying food, wine and shopping opportunities, all in the name of research but we weren't quite sure what for.

To the Pilates of Vero Beach team, especially Camilo A. Rodriguez, my Jiminy Cricket, who makes sure that only the best of my off-the-wall ideas come to fruition, and Eliot Foote. You are the reason I don't have to teach 80 hours a week and could find time to write this book.

My Clara cat, for keeping me sane these last 16 years. When I'm off down a rabbit hole, she's there to remind me that I'm not the only "person" in the world. And by the way, it's time for her shrimp.